"Dawn plays with more veracity than any young pianist I have ever heard. The sublimity of her artistry is mystical."
—Leonard Bernstein

"A memorable memoir about an unforgettable woman who triumphed in the face of adversity. Readers will empathize, sympathize, and care about her. This book is totally unforgettable."
—The Midwest Book Review, Harriet Klausner

"Fascinating . . . deeply impressive . . . an ingenious use of dual perspectives. Dawn Bailiff writes with style and great sensitivity."
—Colin Wilson, author of more than 100 books, including the ground-breaking The Outsider and Beyond the Occult

"Every soul has its own music, and for Dawn Bailiff, it's an ongoing symphony of spirit and power. Her writing style is much like her music . . . driving, insightful, and soulful. Her words will lay open your mind to the great things that can be overcome and accomplished—from the perspective of one who has gone past belief into knowing. Follow her there, for it is the only way to fulfill the promise of life. Notes from a Minor Key will have you majoring in possibility."
—John St.Augustine, author of Living An Uncommon Life and creator/host of Power! Talk Radio

"Bailiff's clarity glistens—and cuts—like ice."
—Chicago Tribune

"Since the time of Job, men have asked: 'Are we on earth to suffer or to be happy?' Dawn Bailiff answers: 'We are here to do both—one does not cancel out the other.' Notes from a Minor Key *is the first-person account—told with cool, relentlessly honest self-appraisal—of someone who has suffered just about every sort of loss imaginable, from her own physical well-being to the people she held dearest, but has miraculously not lost her love of life itself. Her hard-won wisdom is something we would all do well to heed."*
—Gerald Nicosia, author of *Memory Babe: A Critical Biography of Jack Kerouac* and *Home to War*

"Since I have a family member with MS, I understand how much courage it took for Dawn Bailiff to share the details of her illness. Her honest, eloquent portrayal will empower anyone who lives with a chronic illness— and will enlighten anyone who does not."
—Marisa de los Santos, critically acclaimed author of *Love Walked In*

"It is difficult to imagine anyone who wouldn't benefit from this beautifully written and thought-provoking memoir. Dawn Bailiff uses music as a metaphor for life. I highly recommend this book!"
—Greg Schauer, owner of Between Books, Claymont, DE

"Dawn's expression is magical and immediate. Her clear, feminine touch is powerful without being overpowering."
—Sir Georg Solti

"Dawn breathes life into the dead with percussive rhythms that tap into the pulse of life itself. Her passionate life-blood feeds the senses and the soul."
—Carlo Maria Guilini

"Thanks to the sharpness of her fine mind, she navigates the densest landscape with simplicity, bringing clarity to the ambiguous."
—Lorin Maazel

"Bailiff shines her penetrating, singular vision into the heart of the matter. She is a true genius, achieving what all artists hope to achieve but very few do: to uncover the complexity of the simple, to remove all that is unnecessary, to distill the essence of being alive and make it beautiful!"
—Alan Hovhaness

"Dawn Bailiff is simply a natural artist. For her, the level of artistry always comes first, and she is consistently able to sublimate her ego to the higher purpose of her calling. I expect great things from her."
—Shlomo Mintz

"Her interpretation expresses a maturity well beyond her years. Her touch is exquisite, yet powerful. Dare I say, she plays like a man—with the added benefit that she is not a man."
—Daniel Barenboim

"Her amazing gift for melody is only surpassed by her passion—exquisite."
—*Die Welt* (Berlin)

"Thanks to this phenomenal young powerhouse, my view of Chopin has changed forever."
—*Los Angeles Examiner*

"*Like the work of most writers I admire, Bailiff's imagism is hard-edged and direct. I could actually hear the tearing pain in the rhythm of her words. I could even smell the blood.*"
—Carol Gunther, editor of *Protea Poetry Journal*

"*Dawn Bailiff's story is deeply moving and evocative. Her precise and calculated choice of words transports the audience to the waiting room of her diagnosis. Her frustration and isolation as she comes to terms with her illness are real, courageous, and experienced by all who become transformed by the incredible journey of her prose.*"
—Adele Reardon, acquisitions librarian, Bear Public Library, member of American Library Association

"*Reading Dawn Bailiff's* Notes from a Minor Key *not only makes me feel that the world has meaning, but that the world can be healed. She's a writer that needs to be read; she's a writer that influences ideas. Her literary music is a spiritual cry of relief. Nobody less than a genius could have written this book.*"
—D. S. Lliteras, author of *The Master of Secrets*

"*Every life is a story, and yet not every being has the ability or resources to share these events in a cogent way with others. An excellent writer with a marvelous way with words, Dawn Bailiff has overcome great obstacles just to let you read the script her life has written. Read it; you will learn more about yourself.*"
—Jane Reichhold, author of *Writing and Enjoying Haiku: A Hands-On Guide* (Kodansha International)

"Although it was the particular task of my generation of poets to get direct statements of idea back into poetry—after they had been ruled out by Eliot, Pound, and Williams, in favor of concrete detail—only a very few writers can say anything original in terms of idea. Dawn Bailiff is one of those writers."
—W. D. Snodgrass

"Dawn Bailiff's work is in the spirit of the Wise Woman. I could definitely see her work being discussed around the campfires of the future (whatever they might be) as a genuine, honest, voice representing all women of our time."
—J. Greer, editor of *Plains Poetry Journal*

"Edgy, confessional, nervy, dark, honest, spiritual, and validating—there are many words to describe Dawn Bailiff, but 'coward' is certainly not one of them. Her work speaks volumes about debilitating disease, spinning a clear perspective on MS."
—*The News Journal* (Gannett News Service)

notes from a

MINOR KEY

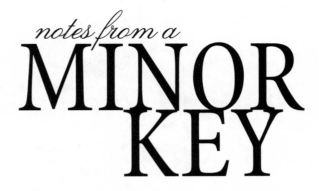

A Memoir of Music, Love, and Healing

DAWN BAILIFF

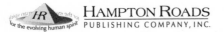

HAMPTON ROADS
PUBLISHING COMPANY, INC.

Cover design by Frame25 Productions
Cover art by iLexx c/o Shutterstock.com, Jaan-Martin Kuusmann c/o
Shutterstock.com, Ariel Schrotter c/o Shutterstock.com, Dan Collier c/o
Shutterstock.com

The poem "Flowers" (Copyright © 1993 by Dawn Bailiff)
originally appeared in *Protea Poetry Journal* (1993).
It was reprinted in *The Poet's Domain,* volume 19 (2002, Live Wire Press)
and again in *Neuroscience Nursing: A Spectrum of Care* by Ellen Barker (2002,
Harcourt/Mosby). Copyright has reverted to author.

Hampton Roads Publishing Company, Inc.
1125 Stoney Ridge Road
Charlottesville, VA 22902

434-296-2772 • fax: 434-296-5096
e-mail: hrpc@hrpub.com • www.hrpub.com

If you are unable to order this book from your local
bookseller, you may order directly from the publisher.
Call 1-800-766-8009, toll-free.

Library of Congress Cataloging-in-Publication Data

Bailiff, Dawn.
Notes from a minor key : a memoir of music, love, and healing / Dawn Bailiff.
p. cm.
Summary: "Dawn Bailiff was a rising star in the classical music world,
performing as a piano soloist with such notable maestros as Leonard
Bernstein and Georg Solti. Then she developed multiple sclerosis. Notes from
a Minor Key tells of her struggle with the debilitating disease and how she
rose from her affliction to become a mother, scholar, and writer"--Provided
by publisher.
ISBN-13: 978-1-57174-554-5 (5.5 x 8.25, tc : alk. paper)
1. Bailiff, Dawn. 2. Pianists--United States--Biography. I. Title.
ML417.B175A3 2007
700.92--dc22
[B]
2007027509

ISBN 978-1-57174-554-5
10 9 8 7 6 5 4 3 2 1
Printed on acid-free paper in the United States

Dedicated to all mothers: may your
heroism no longer be unsung

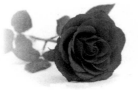

Contents

ATTO II: THE BODY

ATTO III: THE SOUL

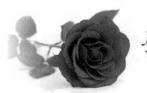

foreword

by D. S. Lliteras

Dawn Bailiff's spiritual memoir, *Notes from a Minor Key,* is possessed by music and passion, intense drama, and heightened imagery. Her prose connects directly to the senses like the impassioned playing of a virtuoso. In fact, I first became acquainted with Dawn Bailiff's artistry through a 1988 recording of her Chopin Preludes, performed at the famed Concertgebouw in Amsterdam when she was in her musical prime as a soloist. Her playing brought me to a new level of understanding, making me listen to music in an entirely different way. I was immediately struck by the percussive, feminine power of her music, and I was deeply moved by her brand of wild and dark passion. I did not know that music could be so personal, so dimensional, so visceral. These are the exact qualities she has translated into her writing, and the result is the very brand of originality and power that most great writers strive for in their work.

Her modern style of storytelling is terse, direct, and engaging, yet she does not sacrifice the classic dramatic form. In fact, even though she writes within structural limitations, she still manages to run wild within these boundaries.

Even more importantly, Dawn Bailiff's *Notes from a Minor Key* has deepened my male understanding and appreciation of a powerful woman's psyche. Her literary perspective is unique because she creates a strong voice that is not apologetic about the female experience. Her fresh and strong perceptions have bridged the gender gap in modern literature: she depicts real women. She is also a brilliant voice in contemporary American literature because her feminine perspective is clear and balanced. She is a writer who influences ideas, who writes with great heart—a writer who needs to not only be read but also experienced. The breath of her feminine voice will not only deepen a woman's consciousness, but will soften a man's recklessness as well. Dare I say, the poignancy of her feminine expression makes me want to be a better man and has certainly deepened my depictions of women in my own work.

For a man, it is rare to get such a clear picture of a woman, seeing her from an increased angle—her desires, her pain, and the effect of her pain upon her. Bailiff is unafraid to show the physicality of womanhood: sexuality, birth—even the blood. In literature, we often get the character of a woman but not her inner workings. *Notes from a Minor Key* shows us both the body and the soul.

Dawn Bailiff has a unique female voice, in that many strong women writers have used men as a benchmark, but Bailiff rejects that paradigm. She brings dignity to women, giving voice to issues that are often not addressed. Women are going to love this book.

Throughout *Notes from a Minor Key,* there runs a spiritual quest that accompanies Dawn's desire to rise in the music world. It is an honest quest to find out where she belongs in the face of

God. Her wisdom is so balanced that I believe her, for she synergizes many spiritual thoughts into a simple wisdom that is grounded in reality. Her bravery is sincere, for her courage is her art. I am grateful that a soul like her exists and that art such as this exists—a memoir equal to great and timeless memoirs of the past, which makes this book literature.

It is important for you to know that Dawn Bailiff wrote this book against all odds; in the face of not only one health problem but many; despite neurological trauma, heavy bleeding, and intense pain. In fact, her extraordinary intellect, her creative power, and her spiritual connectedness have made it possible for her to combat the constant attacks on both her physical and her cognitive abilities by multiple sclerosis. Because most people with her type of advanced condition would be reduced to incompetence and would be unable to function in the most basic way, there are few of us who can truly appreciate how brilliant she has to be in order to conquer these MS attacks.

However, she has transcended the depth of her suffering to become a great woman—musician, wife, and mother—only to lose it all—except for the woman, the powerful woman that she has become, as well as the powerful writer that she is. Were it not for her sheer genius and will, this would not have been possible.

Reading Dawn Bailiff's *Notes from a Minor Key* not only makes me feel that the world has meaning, but that the world can be healed. Her literary music is a spiritual cry of relief in the dark landscape of our time.

D. S. Lliteras
Author of *Jerusalem's Rain* and *The Master of Secrets*

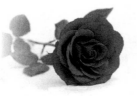

overture

March 2007

As I sit in the oncologist's office, my left leg twitches involuntarily. The doctor has already examined me and my pathology reports, and he looked worried—even nervous—as he excused himself to handle a slight emergency in an adjacent office. My chart is on his desk, so I take the opportunity to sneak a look: "Epithelial undifferentiated ovarian carcinoma, grade three, stage four. Prognosis: Anticipated expiration— three months or less."

In other words, I have ovarian cancer of the most malignant variety, originating from the lining around the ovary and comprised of cells that are difficult to identify. The cancer has already spread to my colon and the lymph nodes in my neck.

Now, most people would be terribly upset upon reading a diagnosis like this, but I merely smile. This is not the first time I have heard it. In fact, I heard the same news five *years* ago! So, I guess I must be doing something right (!) The only reason I am in this office, today, receiving yet another "diagnosis" is because I want an unbiased report to monitor the outcome of my remedies and strategies.

Little does the oncologist know that although my prognosis is bad, I was prepared for it to be even worse. (It can *always* be worse—until it's over; I have learned that.) Little does he know that this news is a relief, for it means I am holding my own. True, my condition has not improved, but more importantly it has not deteriorated as predicted. Had I believed the experts I would have been decomposing in my grave for half a decade by now; instead I am still very much alive—and plan to be for a long time. I know I have everything I need to defeat yet another monster—if "the Big C" only knew what I have triumphed over before meeting up with him . . . Let this beast beware!

Come closer, the Monster will not bite! I have many treasures from my long journey to share with you—many secrets. My journey had three stages: intellectual, physical, and finally, spiritual. It is a tale of healing on all three of these levels. It is also a tale of love. My soul mate, Paul, and I were so close, we almost became one person. So, I cannot tell you my story without showing you his story. Since we were forged together at the time of creation, I am like half a star without him. We are bound like night and day, and you cannot fully comprehend my light without seeing it through his darkness—nor can you bear my darkness without seeing it through his light.

In the end, not only the light—but also the darkness—is a triumph over negative forces. To combat major illness, one must address not only the body, but also the mind and spirit. Damage done to the soul can manifest in physical illness. In order to find healing, one must be prepared to face her demons. Sometimes these demons are where she least expects. I am living proof of this.

I was a prodigy, not only artistically but also psychically. Ironically, my rapid psychic development only served as an impediment to true spirituality. Early in life I learned how to control my environment intellectually, denying my body, which I was later forced to embrace through the challenges of multiple sclerosis. Like the belief that one's soul mate often offers the greatest challenge, instead of the bliss we seek, so goes my relationship with my disability. To find true transformation of my soul, I needed to confront this physical challenge, which I had attempted to deny, to relegate to the *sotto voce* of my life's song.

Why would one be given such talent—musically and psychically—only to have it taken away? Why was I given my self—my identity—so early, when it was that very self that would nearly kill me? These are the questions that *Notes from a Minor Key* seeks to explore, dramatize, and finally, answer.

By bringing me close to death, my physical challenges have brought me closer to life, closer to past life—even closer to future life.

Ignoring a hurting body is a lot like ignoring a crying baby: sooner or later, the abuse will come back to haunt you—and rightfully so.

My pain has been a wake-up call, forcing me to acknowledge the body, which I ignored—denied—for so long in an attempt to achieve intellectual greatness. This new awareness of my body has opened the doors to true spiritual development.

Buddhism teaches that one must master eight steps to achieve enlightenment. The first of these is the ability to see things as they really are. The first step is awareness. Without this, no amount of healing or growth is possible.

Notes from a Minor Key is about coming to one's own spirit through triumph over obstacles. It is about one woman's journey to healing, but it can speak to all of us about how to become whole—whether we are woman or man; whether our challenges are big or small. We are more than our bodies. So much more.

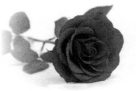

Atto I: THE MIND

Thoughts that breathe and words that burn.
—Thomas Gray

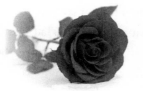

chapter 1: DAWN

December 1986

The keys of the Steinway seemed posed in a smile—the kind that gleams *I wish you well,* while oozing evil intent around the edges. This was the smile that always raised the hairs at the back of my neck, that incited my muscles to pounce . . . that set the butterflies aflutter in my stomach. It was as if this nine-foot monster had its own agenda: to dare me into a sweaty, impassioned set-to, where no weakness was sacred—be it of memory, injury, or anguish.

Softly but deliberately, the orchestra set the syncopated pulse. The opening measures of Mozart's Piano Concerto no. 20 in D Minor washed over Friedberg Hall, filling it with pregnant longing. The uneven groan spoke an uneasiness, which somehow felt inevitable, as though it had always been there—in and around like water.

I awaited my turn to groan, but first my fingers had a new theme to introduce: a playful phrase that danced delightfully in defiance of the brooding that preceded it. Had the despair been real? Had it even existed at all? As if in reply, the orchestra promptly resumed its despondent murmur. This time I was invited to join in—but in an embellished, showy way. Hiding my grief in brilliance as befits the life of the party—the main attraction—I glided around the issue with clever repartee, with slurs as smooth as ice, with arpeggios as perfectly timed as anecdotes. I was at the top of my game . . . and I knew it.

My muscles taut with a passion I did not understand but, like the uneasiness of the music, seemed always to have existed, I merged with the instrument, creating one seamless mass of fingers, wood, and ivory; of strings and blood and bone; of hammers, humidity, and human salts.

I was lost in the music, in the *process,* and it carried me to places unknown—to previously unexplored regions of my mind—and of Mozart's. Dark desire. Pining. Panting.

D minor. Sandwiched between the exuberant expression of the Piano Concerto no. 19 and the no. 21, both written in major keys, Mozart's twentieth piano concerto was a foreshadowing.

The minor key is a place of elemental darkness—of fecundity. *And the earth was without form and void; and darkness was upon the face of the deep.* In this music, the dichotomy of light and dark becomes deeper, facilitating the expansion of the mind. Mozart, who became famous at such a young age by catering to the jovial tastes of Imperial Vienna, seemed to gravitate more to minor keys toward the end of his life. In fact, his Piano Concerto no. 24 in C Minor is a masterpiece of desperate harmonies. Like most geniuses, Mozart anticipated what was to come—the disillusionment with the cerebral abstraction of classical form spawning a revolt to go inward: the Romanticism of the nineteenth century.

Recapitulation. End of the first movement. Cadenza: the technical showcase of the solo instrument. Concentrated, unaccompanied passage work, rounding out the first and final movements of a concerto. Although the cadenzas written by Beethoven for the Mozart 20 fit my fingers well—and were usually a big hit with the tradition-bound judges of these competitions—I went with the ones I had written.

Second movement: the *Romanze*. All the lyrical elegance of well-bred speech, with undertones of resentful fire. The sparks take over, spreading into a passionate interlude that is too short-lived, too desperate. Embers smoldering almost into silence, only to rail once again in mockery: the final movement. *Rondo.* Rapid, rhythmic interchange. An argument of equals. The rondo form is rooted in medieval dance.

My body felt this underlying pulse as a biorhythm, and it responded primitively, rocking with every downbeat.

I had always been told I moved too much onstage. Judges marked down for "extraneous movement." Conductors became . . . distracted. The word "suggestive" had been used to describe my onstage body language more than once. This made little sense to me, being part of a generation raised on rock-and-roll. I was a sixteen-year-old conservatory sophomore with no practical understanding of all those connotations. To me, it was just about the music. Besides, I had always thought that classical musicians could learn a lot from Elvis. . . .

Woodwinds. Trumpets. *Tutti:* The entire orchestra races fervently to a conclusion as if chased by flames, and I am consumed—only to reemerge, triumphant over the fire in a final solo cry of bravura. Man (or, in this case, *Woman*) has won. The concerto ends with . . . enthusiasm.

Yes, that's a good word: from the Greek *entheos* ("in God") although I preferred to think of enthusiasm as being *with* God, in the way that a woman is "with child"—hopeful, fecund, possessed by possibility. To me, being "in God" suggested the peace of certainty, a state of innate knowing, which my intellect did not permit. There was no certainty unmarred by doubt—even in the face of triumph. I sensed that Mozart, in his visceral striving, saw this. Without doubt, there cannot be faith—or determination. It was this determination, inflamed by doubt, that I understood.

It was this determination that had brought me here, to the agonies of turning my art into an athletic spectacle. Well, that and the cash prize. Actually, the year's worth of concert bookings was the real incentive. I had my eye on the future, which made my present pain immaterial. So what if I couldn't afford a decent meal—at least I had a shot at my dream of being a world-class concert pianist.

The Yale Gordon Concerto Competition, held annually at Baltimore's Peabody Conservatory of Music, awarded a top prize of $1,000, a performance with the Peabody Symphony Orchestra, a solo recital in Shriver Hall—on the campus of Peabody's parent University, Johns Hopkins—as well as a series of additional recitals scheduled by the Peggy and Yale Gordon Trust. Winning this competition offered a lot of bang for the buck, and despite the fact that my performance credentials were already considered impressive, I wanted the exposure. Baltimore was, after all, my hometown, and even after receiving college admission to Peabody (one of the top three music conservatories in the U.S.) at the age of fifteen, I still felt underappreciated in this dark city, nestled around the Inner Harbor like a brooding panther.

It was difficult to assert oneself, lest the panther strike. In many ways, I had become invisible, vapid among the dirty streets of blue-collar minutiae. But the focus of mere survival was strangely comforting, even as it threatened to strangle; I wanted out.

The sound of applause wooed me from my reverie, and my gaze traveled around the marble and gold of the Miriam A. Friedberg Concert Hall. Gods, seraphim, and other mythologically perfect beings seemed to glare down from icy pillars. I quickly reminded myself that this blatant homage to Old World architecture was atoned for by modern stage lighting, multi-track recording equipment, and an orchestra pit with hydraulic lift.

Most of the 800 seats were filled, but the acoustics prevented the roar from swallowing me up, as had happened in some halls. I never liked the sound of applause; it always made me feel vulnerable, exposed, even a little silly—like prancing around in one's underwear for approval.

I was overheated from the physical and emotional effort of the music, and my floor-length, long-sleeved black velvet did not help. Imagining a trail of sweat following me like bread crumbs to mark my path, I made my way backstage to await the verdict. Luck had prevailed to give me the enviable last performance slot, which meant my impact would be longer and my wait, shorter.

Nonetheless, it was still a wait—and a weighty wait at that. Scenes of my first visit to the Friedberg overtook my nervous mind: a small child, five or six, already musically gifted, escorted by my mother to the Tuesday noon recital series to hear Peabody's future stars perform. At the time, names had meant nothing to me, so the raw purity of body and mind had been mine to enjoy.

There had been another element, a powerful presence in the hall that had off-centered my young nerves in a way I could not yet understand.

Years later, during my first day as a conservatory student, I stepped into the Friedberg once again. Tears filled my eyes as I experienced, in an instant, the cumulative force of creative energy that seemed to radiate from the walls. I could feel the presence of all the greats who had come before me: Tchaikovsky, Stravinsky— even Ralph Waldo Emerson had once graced this stage. I believed in the eternity of their creations and felt, as did Isaac Newton, that "I stood on the shoulders of giants."

My wait was over. Jonathan Gold, a junior, won. I came in second: $350—and that was it. No recital, no bookings. Second place may sound impressive, but it is a lot like winning first runner-up at the Miss America Pageant: no one pays any attention. By the way, at the Yale Gordon Concerto Competition, there is no third prize . . .

Backstage, I unhooked my long braid from around my head, changed into a denim skirt, and reluctantly threw on an oversized sweater to protect my overheated body from the December cold. After slipping my feet into my well-worn Docksiders, I bundled my performance gear into an equally worn black suitcase and gave the lid a hard shove, more from frustration than necessity. The curt finality of the lock's *snap* seemed all too appropriate. Although held annually, the Yale Gordon rotates each year in the disciplines of strings, orchestral instruments, and piano and is open only to students of the Peabody Conservatory. Since pianists would not be permitted to compete for another three years, and I was already a sophomore, this was my last chance at first prize. Who would've thought that a bloodless tight-ass like Gold could win with that staid, banal rendition of the Saint-Saëns Second? I clicked my tongue across my teeth in disgust. Now in street clothes, I was reduced to your basic urban teenager—nothing to emulate; something, perhaps, to be feared. Although I was tiny enough to look more like twelve than sixteen, years of *tae kwon do* had made me wiry. Well, I had needed to be strong: the city streets where I had grown up were no safe place for a half-Jewish, half-Japanese runt of a girl who happened to play the piano.

In my present set of circumstances, it seemed that my strength would continue to be called upon. The year was 1986, and there was little room in the yuppie society for edgy, nonmaterialistic youth.

Emerging, deep in thought, from the stage door, I was blindsided by a nervous young man. His speech was rapid and effusive, his eyes, intense and engaging. "I can't believe they gave first prize to that musical turd," he gushed. "That guy plays it way too safe . . . You positively blew him off the stage . . . Anybody could see that. You were fire and ice! By the way, I'm Paul Bailiff. I never knew Mozart could . . . evoke such . . . dark passion."

I mustered a weak half-smile—probably one of my most cynical—as I turned to give him the once-over. Close to a foot taller than I, he was quite thin but appeared strong. His hair, which he wore short, in classic Cary Grant style, was blue-black—like mine. His ears stuck out slightly, pleasantly. Square, well-defined jaws supported the tight temples and knotted brow that, in turn, capped truly magnificent eyes. His eyes, shielded behind small wire-framed glasses, were also black. He was definitely cute.

"Dark passion?" I probed. "Is that your area of expertise?"

"Uhhh . . . let's just say, I am familiar with the concept." He blushed slightly, then looked away.

Oh. Perhaps I had been a bit too probing. "Well, thank you," I said with reservation. "It's nice to be appreciated . . . Too bad you're not one of the judges. Now if you'll excuse me, before I collapse, I need to go home to my bassoon-playing roommate from hell. Well actually, she's from Minnesota."

"Is there a difference?" he retorted.

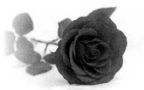

chapter 2: PAUL

January 1987

Cat piss or stale beer? I was trying to figure out the smell coming from the battered sofa in Gina's apartment, when she rounded the corner from the small kitchen and handed me a bottle of suds. Heaving a sigh, which seductively shifted her large breasts, she said, with more concern than the situation seemed to warrant, "Don't worry, Paul, if you spill the beer; it's happened many times before."

Like I cared.

"Well, you'd never know it," I replied, with full knowledge that I, Paul Bailiff, would not be the first guy to score on this couch.

"I shouldn't do this with my roommate asleep in the bedroom but here goes," Gina continued, giggling softly. She removed a record from its battered sleeve and placed it on the turntable. The opening strains of Fauré's Piano Quartet no. 1 breathed life into the stagnant air. Delicately sensual as the composer's native tongue of French, the melody did, for me, what the beer could not: ease that damned anxiety. Delicately sensual. *That's* what a woman should be: silk, not sandpaper . . . We had just bought the record that day—used.

"Hmmm . . . I wanna write a piece like this," she cooed, nestling against me. Gina was a composition major at the Peabody, as was I.

"Don't strive to create what's already been created," I said. "Write something better."

"Uhhh, figures you'd say that, Mr. *Definitive-Work-That-Cannot-Be-Surpassed,*" she groaned, referring to my favorite George Bernard Shaw quote. "What kind of a goal is that anyway? If other artists have not created the definitive work, how can you or I? . . . How can you not like this piece just the way it is?"

"You're missing the point," I replied, attempting to hide my frustration. "The quest for the definitive work is an individual matter; it's about scaling your own heights, not measuring your climb against someone else's . . . Anyway, I love this piece—as Fauré. It wouldn't work as Gina Strippone."

"You're such a hypocrite." She smiled mischievously. "The only reason you like this piece is because it has the influence of your buddy Schumann all over it!"

I shrugged in silence because it was true. The manic desperation of Robert Schumann's music had always seemed to speak to me, alone—like he and I had some kind of private understanding. I was never sure, though, how much was the music, itself, and how much was my identification with his madness.

"Oh, there it is," Gina chided as she curled her index finger into a girlish point, "that mad, brooding composer stance! That's one advantage you male artists have: the more ill-tempered and off-center you are, the more the world fears and respects you. If we women try to pull that crap, we're just labeled crazy bitches!"

"Either that or you must have PMS," I added flatly, hoping to put her on the defensive. As much as I disliked Gina's cerebral aggression, I was actually relishing the distraction from her physical brashness. Gina's tirades about how PMS was really a myth, used by men and weak females to keep women second-class, were well-known. Unfortunately, she refused to be diverted.

"You're incorrigible," Gina sighed as she began to nibble on my ear. She had already finished her beer, while I had taken barely a swig from mine. The smell of alcohol was all over her: a definite turnoff. It reminded me of my mother.

"The thing is, you men always need a strong yet nurturing woman to help you reach your 'definitive work,'" Gina whispered seductively while stroking my chest, her cheekbone resting against my shoulder. "Even Schumann had Clara Wieck . . . I could be *your* Clara Wieck."

I gently fingered her pointed chin to turn her face toward mine, to look into her feisty brown eyes. "You're forgetting one thing," I started gently. "Clara Wieck was a staid, cool, cerebral German, who lived in complete subordination to her husband, having his babies and interpreting his music. Although a talented writer, she never got the chance to be a composer in her own right, constantly living in his shadow—even after he went mad. You're a hot-blooded, opinionated Mediterranean with a keen eye on your own career. You'd never be satisfied deferring to a man for any reason."

"Except for love," she shot at me with glaring eyes.

"Ah, but don't you see? That's the worst reason of all . . ."

She seemed to ponder my words, sighing in resignation as her practical bent took over: there was simply no point in pursuing this. Settling back against my chest, she unbuttoned the top two buttons of my shirt so as to slide her hand inside, caressing my skin, playing with the hairs on my chest the way girls do.

Stroking her shiny black hair, her neck, her back, I took a moment to reflect on the absurdity of Gina's comparing herself to Clara Wieck. The pictures I had seen of Schumann's wife had shown her to be pale, thin, angular; gentle and patient; quietly strong. The insecurity of perfectionism was all over her. Gina, on the other hand, was olive-skinned, voluptuous; impetuous, full of bravado and herself. Clara Wieck was a lot more like . . . like that pianist I had seen before winter break in the Yale Gordon; that pianist whose artistic presence had rendered me into such a spastic basket case I couldn't even talk to her like a normal person. She probably thought I was really strange, going on about *fire and ice* and *dark passion* . . . Dawn. What was her last name? It was a German name . . . Wasserman? . . . No . . . Wassmer! That's it. Dawn Wassmer, with her dark braid wrapped around her head in antiquated fashion, her ivory skin, her intense blue eyes. Quiet strength exuded from her—and from her music. She clearly understood the reticence of perfectionism.

Was she beautiful? I honestly didn't know. What's more, her power over me was already so great, I didn't care . . .

Gina could be considered beautiful—well actually, cute was more like it: cute in a seductive way. Her rounded, rosy features reminded me of the Kewpie doll I had won throwing darts for my first girlfriend in high school. Yet, Gina was all woman—no good little girl here—if you define "good" as being asexual. She was certainly a good person: considerate, generous, concerned, and attentive toward those she loved. And she loved me. This made her difficult to resist. Too bad she was so aggressive. Call me old-fashioned, but I liked the uncertainty of the pursuit, the fantasy that mystery afforded. Gina's low-cut sweater with push-up bra left little to the imagination. Also, she seemed a bit too comfortable making the first move. I suddenly realized that I would rather not go where so many men had gone before. As her hand clasped the back of my neck, pulling my face to her lips, I wondered why I was even here. As her hand teased my crotch, I remembered the reason: Gina knew exactly what to do . . . Just then, a loud buzzer sounded.

"Oh, shoot," Gina hissed as her body became tense. "That's the downstairs security door. Maybe they'll go away."

Two more buzzes in quick succession.

"Ohhh," moaned Gina as she rose from the couch, feigning pain. "That must be Christina's boyfriend; he always rings right together like that." She walked over to a cumbersome-looking intercom attached to the side wall and pressed the door-release button.

"Shouldn't you find out who it is first?" I asked, pointing to the speaker.

"Naw, I know it's Joe. Don't worry; he won't bother us. He'll just go in with Christina." She nodded toward the bedroom. "Hey, Sleeping Beauty! Your smoochy babe is here!" She projected like an opera star, then turned to open the apartment door.

Peering down the hallway (perhaps she wasn't so sure it was Joe after all), her back suddenly stiffened in what seemed to be surprise. "Hey, girlfriend! How the hell *are* you?" Gina's voice echoed through the hallway as the visitor emerged. I couldn't believe my eyes.

"Paul, I'd like you to meet my friend, Dawn Wassmer."

Rising from the couch, I held out my hand: "Pleased to meet you."

"Dawn, this is Paul Bailiff. He's a junior in the Composition Department."

"Very nice to meet you, Paul." Dawn took my hand and gave it a firm squeeze. Not surprisingly, she had glorious hands: small yet long-fingered and slender; graceful yet strong. I felt a strange sensation as our hands met for that fraction of a moment, like our souls had interacted before. As we released our grip, the residue of centuries of feeling stretched between us. Did she recognize me? I could not tell.

Gina turned to Dawn: "What are you doing out so late?"

"Just walking."

"Just walking?" Gina repeated incredulously. "Alone? . . . In this neighborhood? . . . In the freezing cold?"

"I like the cold," replied Dawn, rubbing her hands together. "And I'm *from* the inner city, remember? Besides, I really did have a mission—earlier: I went to make copies." She patted the black canvas bag that was strapped over her shoulder.

"Copies?" Gina and I asked in unison.

"Yeah, I had to photocopy my score to submit to the chair of the Opera Department and his committee. Then I was so stressed about the whole situation that I just went walking—until I ended up here." She turned to Gina: "I didn't realize you had company. If I'm in the way, I can leave . . . we can always talk tomorrow . . ."

"Not a chance," Gina breathed with excitement. "I wanna hear what the hell you're doing with the Opera Department— and why you're so stressed." Her eyes darted in my direction, scanning for objections. I just shrugged in an attempt to appear nonchalant.

"Well, okay then," Dawn said definitively as she quickly removed her tattered coat and flung it on the back of the wicker chair in which she then sat. Gina and I resumed our positions on the couch directly across from Dawn. Christina, who had just stumbled into the living room, looking confused, nodded sleepily to Dawn and perched herself upon the arm of the couch without saying a word.

"I submitted my opera to Randy Fetzer—you know, the student rep," Dawn proceeded rapidly, gesturing with her hands. "Anyway, he loved it. He said I had an 'amazing gift for melody,' but he was unwilling to recommend my work for performance because I am not a composition major. Further, he told me that no composition majors have submitted operas this year for performance, and—since the budget allows for one student opera production a year—they are trying to recruit a composition student to write an opera. Can you believe it? The guy actually loves my work, and he *still* won't recommend me? So, I'm going in front of the committee myself: it's a stupid rule, and someone needs to challenge it."

"Wait a minute," Gina interjected. "You wrote an opera? An entire opera? Who wrote your libretto?"

"I wrote it myself," Dawn stated matter-of-factly. "It is based on a short story I wrote in high school. It's called *Biancola*—about a girl by that name. You see, she goes into the woods to kill herself—to hang herself—but she doesn't succeed. Instead of dying, she finds God."

I glanced self-consciously at the scars on my wrists.

"You have a copy of the score," I said, nodding toward her bag. "May we see it?"

"Sure." Dawn gingerly removed the thick score and handed it to me as though it were made of porcelain.

"She acts like it's her baby doll," Christina teased as if reading my mind.

"Worse than that: it's her *newest* baby doll," Gina explained, exchanging with me a knowing look. Only another composer could understand the overprotective angst surrounding a manuscript—copy or no. A singer like Christina simply could not.

The three of us, hovering in a half circle, pored over the pages like kids over a treasure map—but this music was no kids' stuff. Chords crashed to the caverns of darkness; melodies soared to the higher reaches of the soul. Life ended, only to be reborn. One phrase melted inevitably into the next as the human voice became a vehicle for the spirit—for the part of us that has no limitations.

"Hey, this is awesome!" Christina's voice broke the intensity of the silence. "Can I sing the soprano lead?"

Dawn just smiled at that. It was a nice smile—gentle and girlish. The brilliance of her smile made it difficult to pull myself back to the score.

The brilliance of her score made it even more difficult to find something to criticize. The orchestration was tight, and the tonality was so complex I couldn't figure it out. Yet, everything simply worked in such a way that the suggestion of change would be difficult. Her knowledge of the individual instruments was impeccable: each orchestral part was so suited to the strengths and idiosyncrasies of its instrument that it seemed improvised.

I needed to find something seemingly constructive to say about this seemingly effortless work in order to restore balance in myself. This was written by a pianist—a mere interpreter—not even a member of the Composition Department. I was a serious composition student, but the work did not come easily to me.

The desire to become a composer began to stir in me at about age twelve; however, not coming from a musical family, I didn't know what to do about it. Short stints with a series of teachers—in both piano and composition—yielded little. In what felt like a counterattack, I spent many a Saturday at the

University of Washington Library poring over weighty texts of music theory, counterpoint, and orchestration. Teaching myself enough French and German to get by and also to play a mean— if mechanical—piano rounded out my cultural education.

Through all of this, the darkness chewed at my sense of being like an obscene monster, taking sadistic pleasure in my torment. Despite threats to the contrary, my body remained alive; only my mind was in tatters—uncertain, indecisive. After graduating from high school, I floundered around for two years, trying to find my voice. Strictly as a long shot, I contacted Peabody in late spring, fairly certain there would be no available slots for the upcoming fall. To my surprise, one of the previously accepted students had decided to study in Europe, so there was still a slot in the Composition Department. But what could I do—a self-taught twenty-year-old with no major teacher behind him—to impress one of the top conservatories in the world, a school used to having thirteen-year-old prodigies practically begging for admission? I did what any stubborn, idealistic artist would do: I worked like hell. I worked like my life depended on it—which, of course, it did. For three weeks, I slaved with almost no sleep to write my *Piano Concerto for a Dying Man.* That's what I called it because everything I had been was at war with everything I wanted to become: part of me had to die to allow the rest of me to live. I was going under, and this was my only way out, this music that had the potential to save me.

Now, music, again, held this power. The darkness and doubt I had always felt were reflected in Dawn's opera. But there was something else. The voice of God called to me, through this universal language, reminding me I was not alone, that there were others on the same journey. Had Dawn been through the same crisis of faith as had I? She certainly knew enough to write about it. I was suddenly assured the emotions I had felt at the Friedberg that December afternoon had not been misplaced: this was my soul mate, sitting close enough to touch.

Yet, what could I do? I was with Gina, a girl who was very into me and had done nothing to deserve ill treatment. And yet, how could I allow this opportunity to slip through my fingers: perhaps my one chance at real happiness? And yet again, how can one be truly happy knowing one's happiness came at the expense of someone else?

The Rodgers and Hammerstein song "This Nearly Was Mine" played in my brain as I wondered why life, so much of the time, was based on near misses. Entire lifetimes were made or broken on hairline fractures of choice or chance.

. . . They told me that I almost didn't get in, that I gained admission to Peabody solely based on the strength of my piano concerto. . . .

At the same moment, Gina and I looked up from the score, and our eyes met. Without speaking, we knew what the other one was thinking: *Wow!* The music superseded all else. This was clearly the work of a mature artist.

"My work was nothing like this when I was a sophomore," Gina, now a junior, sighed.

"What do you mean?" Dawn asked quickly.

"It just wasn't." Gina's lips tightened, and I could see the jealousy in her eyes. Still, she refused to be made small by this emotion. Turning to me, she fished: "You've collaborated with Randy, couldn't you help her?" A clever maneuver to make herself look benevolent without having to be so: she knew that Randy and I had had a serious falling-out. I refused to take the bait.

"I'll certainly see what I can do," I stated confidently without looking either woman in the eyes. Gina shrugged as she stood up from the couch.

"That would be great," Dawn said softly.

I suspected that Dawn, with her high intelligence, had been able to figure out what had just transpired, so I was appreciative of her allowing my graceful escape.

"Would anybody like a beer?" Gina called from the kitchen.

"Yeah, I'll take one," Christina yelled, even though the kitchen was not that far away.

"No, thank you," I responded.

"How about you, Dawn?" Gina called back.

Dawn, who had seemed to be waiting to see what I would do, replied: "No—thanks anyway, Gina—I really should be getting home. I have a long day tomorrow—and a long walk tonight." She packed up her score, picked up her coat, then added with a tinge of embarrassment: "I live in the dorm."

"What a coincidence," I chimed in as I stood to help her with her coat. "Since I reside there myself, why don't I walk you home?"

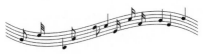

"Of course I remember." Dawn placed the third and fourth fingers of her left hand across her lips in a moment of contemplation. "'What man art thou, that, thus bescreen'd in night, so' . . . studiest dark passions?" Her voice had a mischievous tone.

"You're a devil," I said playfully. "I honestly couldn't tell if you remembered me or not."

"Sooo, does that mean I am hard to read—a woman of mystery?"

"On the contrary, I believe I can read you quite well . . . at least, on important matters."

"And what might they be?" She asked coquettishly, batting her eyes.

Feeling a little weak in the knees, I stopped walking and turned my full attention on her. The January cold had brought a splash of color to her otherwise pale cheeks, which served as an appropriate backdrop to the childish curiosity dominating her heart-shaped face. Although she wore no make-up, she looked like a delicately painted china doll: flawless. Her eyes were impelling. Should I answer? I thought it best to wait.

Baltimore's Mount Vernon District has five blocks of antique stores and at least one hundred shops; so, what were our chances of walking past the very shop where Gina and I had bought that Fauré record? Nonetheless, there we were. Dawn actually stopped to look inside the store window. Eerily, she turned to me and asked with curious innocence: "Do you think Gina will hate me, I mean, since we left her apartment together?"

Another question I thought it best not to answer.

We continued along North Charles Street toward the Conservatory, passing some of the most unique buildings in Baltimore.

Unlike the cookie-cutter trend in modern construction, the townhouses and brownstones dominating the Mount Vernon District—named after George Washington's Virginia planta-tion—reflect the eclectic tastes of post-Civil War aristocrats. Greek and Renaissance Revival, Beaux Arts, and Georgian archi-tecture coexist harmoniously in their differences in a way that people, themselves, cannot.

At long last, I broke the silence with a question of my own: "If you have enough craft to write an entire opera, why aren't you in the Composition Department?"

"I've been a pianist all of my life—and not much else. Composers are supposed to be more . . . sophisticated . . . more erudite."

"Is that so?" I asked in slight amusement.

She began to blush. "I mean that I never had the time to become that well-rounded, to figure out literary allusions for the names of my pieces or to understand what's so great about the twelve-tone system. Music, for me, has always been much more about, well, just doing it, so to speak, about practicing, raw expression—about passion."

"That may be," I started carefully, "but you must still be a fairly well-rounded person to write an opera that deals with spirituality, myth, philosophy—not exactly the product of someone who has spent her life mindlessly banging away at the keys."

"Maybe it has nothing to do with the mind." She smiled wryly. "Maybe it's just about courage—or lack of courage. Composers need the courage to persuade others: to perform their music, to listen to an idea that has never existed before. The ability to turn the abstract into the tangible boils down to networking. Besides, it's difficult to be the only girl in a department full of guys—just ask Gina."

There was a determination in Dawn's eyes that made it difficult to imagine her without courage. Still, I could appreciate what she meant. Composition was certainly a male-centric discipline—and there was nothing masculine about Dawn. She seemed unapologetic in her femininity, without trying to use it to her advantage. I would expect that a girl like that could feel invisible among the intellectually brazen egotists of the Composition

Department. Nonetheless, it was still an enigma how someone as extraordinary as Dawn could be so insecure, so unaware of her greatness.

"You shouldn't deny yourself opportunities because of a silly little obstacle like people," I quipped.

"Silly little obstacle? You're crazy," she giggled lightly. "Anyway, not only would I be the next-to-the-only girl in the Composition Department, I'd also be the youngest member. I'm sixteen."

Sixteen! Whoa. I would turn twenty-three in March.

"Anyway," she continued, "I'm almost too old to break into that final top tier as a concert artist—the blue-hairs only want to buy tickets to see the cute little twelve-year-olds perform Rachmaninov's Second as though they were shaking water from their fingertips. If I really want to do this, it's now or never. I can't believe it has already been four years since I was one of those twelve-year-olds—and I *was* a hit back then. When I was thirteen, I did a twelve-city tour across Europe, and both the audiences and the critics loved me. *Die Welt* called my playing 'exquisite,' and *The London Times* said that my 'tiny fingers evoked magic.' Can you believe it? And I was paid a lot, too! I also played in Japan, Hong Kong, Korea, all over South America, and other places I can't remember. My father dragged me around the world like a traveling salesman, which, I guess, in a way, he was . . . selling *me!*" Her face knotted in frustration.

"Look," I said gently, "from what I heard last month, you don't need anybody to sell you; your talent will sell itself."

"That's sweet, however naïve." She smiled wryly. "*Every*thing has to be sold. Nothing is good enough to sell itself. The world only seeks what is shoved down its throat." Her tone suddenly became mysterious: "I have a need to perform now, while my physical powers are at their zenith, before it's too late—I can't explain that. It is just a sense I have. There will be time later to compose, to be intellectually fecund. I can hear the music in my head that I will someday create."

So there was some confidence after all . . . hearing music in her head. I envied musicians who could do that. A layer had always existed between my self and the printed sheet of music. I knew what I was looking at, for sure, but it was an intellectual process, a knowledge of what it *should* sound like. I did not know how to bring in the sound, to sense it on the cellular level. Dawn's powers suddenly struck me in a way I could not have anticipated, dousing my ego like a bucket of ice water. She was actually choosing from among her talents, not to be ruled by one, solitary gift, the way I was. A female like this perplexed me, for, although I had never actually operated on the presumption that women were intellectually inferior, I had, nonetheless, always found them to be so. This was simply not true of Dawn.

As we approached Mount Vernon Place—the square facing Peabody—none other than George Washington stared us down from the height of a 178-foot classic Greek Doric column. The pristine quality of this spotlighted monument in marble—the first one in the nation erected to him—shone as incongruously against the city smog as a candle in a bowl of pea soup. The four parks that flanked the monument were also incongruous: addicts, hookers, and sundry street folks defied the pretense of Euro-elegance that the fountains and flowers would suggest. A sense of gritty desperation made it hard to believe that this area had once been sought after by society's elite, that climbers like F. Scott Fitzgerald had actually called Mount Vernon home.

Nonetheless, the Peabody itself painted an impressive picture. Completed in 1866 by the English architect, Edmund Lind, the original conservatory—where classes were still held—had been built in the Renaissance Revival style, replete with winding staircases, arched windows, and carved entablatures. The contrast provided by the stark, modern complex, situated to the south, that housed the cafeteria, garage, and dormitories, created a kind of gestalt of past and present. The continuum of change always made me feel eerie—like riding a glass elevator to the top of a fifty-story building: although you're fairly confident of the outcome, the trip itself is disconcerting.

We came first to Schapiro House, as it faces on North Charles Street. The sight of this mid-nineteenth century townhouse always made me a little tense, for this was the home of the school's administrative offices. I had never been there except to straighten out some bureaucratic bull—time I could not spare and would never recoup; time I needed to spend on my music.

"Hey, can you spare seventy-five cents so's I can buy a loaf of bread?" a disheveled man slurred, coming so close I could smell the cheap wine on his breath.

"No, we can't; we work for what we get," Dawn snapped, glaring fearlessly at the man, who began to glare back. We escaped through the security gate into a dingy alley that led to the heart of the concrete campus.

"Did you know that Peabody was modeled after Paris' *Conservatoire de Musique?*" I asked.

"Yes, and it's fitting, considering that Peabody was the first music conservatory to be founded in America, and the *Conservatoire* was the first conservatory of the modern world," she replied.

"That's a remarkable fact to have at your fingertips," I quipped.

"Well, I have a brain for useless facts."

"Maybe they're not so useless," I replied.

"I always wanted to attend the Paris *Conservatoire*," she continued. "Guiomar Novaës, the Brazilian pianist, graduated from there with first prize; she was my idol when I was little. I remember the first time I heard her play. I was about eight when I checked out a recording of hers from the public library: three of the Beethoven sonatas. One of them was the *Moonlight*, which I had been working on all that summer. What I heard was so wild, so different from anything I had ever heard before." Dawn's eyes began to glisten as her hands gestured creatively. "The only interpretations of Beethoven I had heard, up to that point, had been from men—and I didn't understand them. Guiomar's playing was powerful and gentle at the same time, so unapologetically female with its percussive passion." By now, Dawn's eyes positively shone, and her face glowed with excitement. God, she was beautiful. I was certain of that now. Despite the cold, my body began to feel too warm.

I cleared my throat. "So why didn't you go to Paris?" I asked, more for a distraction than anything else.

"My father wanted me to stay—he needs me, I guess. My mother died when I was twelve. I have two older sisters—quite a bit older—so they already have their own lives . . . husbands, kids, and all that. My father and I have always had a special bond. My mother and I were never that close." Her face winced in memory.

"My mother never had much use for me, except when I was playing the piano. Well, I really was pretty uncoordinated away from the instrument—still am." There again was that wry smile. "Anyway, I remember one time, when I was about six, helping my mother in the kitchen. There was a big, orange ceramic bowl that my mother really liked. Well, I was carrying it from the kitchen to the dining room table and—*splat!* I simply lost control of my hands and, in an instant, the entire kitchen was covered with pasta salad. It was garnished, if you will, with orange slivers—and I don't mean the fruit. I had barely processed what had happened when—*whack!*—my mother backhanded me with so much force I fell flat on my *tochis*. My father, who was sitting at the dining room table, quietly set down the newspaper he'd been reading, stood up, walked over to my mother—just as quietly—and slapped her in the face. Then, he said sternly but calmly: 'Don't hit her in the face anymore.' No kidding!"

After studying my countenance for a moment, Dawn suddenly looked embarrassed. "You probably think I'm crazy, talking about my parents that way, but I find you're really easy to talk to. I don't usually open up like this. . . . Actually, it was the only time I ever saw my father hit my mother."

"It's all right," I reassured her. "I'm not that close to my mother either."

We proceeded to the dormitory, and I walked her to her door. "Well, I guess I'll see you around," she whispered nervously as her eyes quickly scanned the hallways.

"Yeah," I whispered back. "I'd rather not get caught in the girls' dormitory—yet I couldn't just leave you at the elevator." I handed her bag, which I had been carrying, back to her.

She fumbled nervously for her keys, erasing all surreptitious efforts with the loud thud of her bag dropping against the concrete floor. Books of all shapes, sizes, and colors scattered and lay flat, like dying insects. The book that grabbed my attention, however, was a tattered trade paperback with a bright yellow backdrop, supporting the bold blue title: *Your Psychic Powers and How to Develop Them* by Hereward Carrington. I had come across this spiritualist classic in my early teens and had been inexplicably drawn to it—then repelled by it. It seemed that Dawn was even more interesting than I had thought—and more frightening.

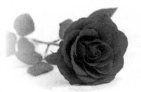

chapter 3: DAWN

February 1987

Groaning cellos, chirping flutes, and desperate pianos threatened to drown out my inner voice as I sat on the hard wooden bench in the hall of the conservatory. Sketching a flute sonata that I wanted desperately to finish for my good friend and brilliant flautist, Amy Hagaman, by tomorrow, I tried to push thoughts of Paul from my mind. This was a bit too much to expect of myself, considering that I sat about two feet from the closed door of the practice studio he was currently occupying. The studio door had a glass pane at the top, so I could see Paul's head bobbing up and down at the piano. I could even—when he cocked his head to one side—see his mouth form a determined grimace as he quickly jotted down what he had discovered.

It was a strange comfort to be near him, even though we were on tenuous terms. Our meeting at Gina's had only been a few weeks ago, but the intensity between us that evening had made me presume . . . something. Not that we hadn't spent a great deal of time together—having coffee, hanging out in the practice rooms, walking the Inner Harbor or Little Italy, always talking, talking. It seemed that we never ran out of things to say to one another. One night we actually spent eight hours just talking. There was just a certain coolness, a certain holding back that had definitely developed after that first night. This confused me, and I was not easily confused about such things. Since earliest memory, I have always had a kind of sixth sense about people— their motives, their feelings, even their pasts. I had a sense of something in Paul's past that was very dark. This darkness attracted me to him.

Psychically, I was already sufficiently linked to him to have an awareness of where he might be at any given moment. Most of the time, I was right—as I had been this evening. The number "3" had kept popping into my mind, dancing across Paul's long, powerful fingers. Symbols. You gotta love 'em. Sure enough, there he was in *studio 3,* using those fingers to pull music from his mind.

Unlike Paul, I did not need a piano to compose. This gave me the freedom to actually get some work done, while enjoying a strategic view. If only I had the courage to simply walk over, knock on the door, and address Paul directly, unleashing all the ambivalence now locked inside my heart. Still, I had another option.

The first time I had been able to project my psyche was at the age of seven, during an attack of rheumatic fever. Pain radiated from all my joints and from my temples. The heat inside was so intense, my brain felt like it was cooking. All of a sudden, I began to gradually disconnect from my body, clicking off like a string of tiny light switches. Then, I felt a powerful surge, as I was pushed forth from my flesh in one gigantic wave—kinda like being born, I guess, except I was free—free from the heat, free from the pain. I didn't go very far that first time, floating above my body like I was obliged to watch over it. Later, however, I learned that, with effort, I could travel anywhere I could imagine.

Now, the only place I could imagine was with Paul. My eyes scanned for a private space: someone was just leaving a studio at the end of the hall. I quickly assembled my belongings and seized the room. Locking the door behind me, I settled into a well-worn, upholstered chair against the back wall.

Slowly, I transferred my awareness to successive points along my physical form, consciousness reflecting into the etheric body. Centering my will into a single force of energy, I propelled my consciousness into *studio 3*. It felt so good to be in Paul's presence, experiencing him in his "natural state," so to speak: the full reflection of his self-awareness. Since human consciousness is a cocktail of objective activity and subjective fantasy, I could, being in the astral dimension, view Paul's tangible existence and his thought-life simultaneously. Like abstract photography, disjointed images blurred together in the echoes of experience. In the foreground was a slightly older, more distinguished Paul on the conductor's podium, exuding artistry and confidence. The background contained little Paul, at the age of four, cowering in the corner, his face distorted by fear. Between these two images was Paul at his present age, but with a demeanor much more dejected than I could normally perceive. He appeared deflated against the keyboard, his head in his right hand, blue-sleeved elbow propped against the shiny black, his eyes a little too intent upon the left hand, crawling across the keys. Sometimes, he grimaced; sometimes, he sighed. He seemed kind of pathetic, sitting there. I wanted to comfort him, an act for which I would not have the courage in my physical state, to envelop him in the gentleness of my soul. But wait a minute! I was annoyed with him: why was he distancing himself from me, keeping me at arm's length? Supposedly, I was here to find some answers. And yet, frustrated and confused as I was, it was difficult to remain angry in his presence, difficult to believe in my doubts. I felt so complete with him that the desire to simply enjoy the moment drowned out the darkness. I knew that the darkness would return soon enough—as soon as I was alone again. Paul was a match, lighting a candle in my soul—a warm glow that was snuffed out the moment he left.

Was this love? I didn't know. I only knew that I had never felt this way before. What's more, I didn't like it. I felt like a stone about to face the sculptor's chisel. Then I recalled how the *Zohar*, the major text of Kabbalah, described the relationship between soul mates as one of "correction" of the soul, brought about not by bliss but through challenge. Soul mates are two halves of a whole, and the welding together of these two halves can be painful. I understood and accepted the necessity—even the value—of pain, but this did not prevent my disliking it.

Despite my dislike, this pain would connect me to him. Of that, I was certain.

As if in response to my faith, another aspect of Paul's consciousness became perceptible: his image of me. I could actually see myself being seen. It was as if I had become the art and the onlooker, the beauty and the beholder, simultaneously. There were various shadows of me, each more beautiful than I had ever been, more benevolent, more gentle. What he saw in me was far greater than anything I could see in myself. How could I live up to his expectations? How could I be deserving? What should have made me happy felt like a tremendous weight upon my soul. I felt myself drained into transparency by the power of his conception. It was exhilarating—but even more frightening. Frightening because I could feel my true self evaporating: I needed the freedom to be the imperfect being that I was—or I could not be at all. I needed my darkness in order to become light. How could he see me without seeing me?

In his impressions, I also looked younger than I felt, more girlish, more innocent—childlike even. Yet, I was eerily wise: a tiny creature with a huge brain, an intellect worthy of a sci-fi thriller, sucking all the life from the feeble body that supports it. Is that what I was to him—some kind of lopsided *enfant terrible?* Not the complete woman I wanted to be.

I needed him to know me without the pretensions of my flesh; yet, when he finally looked in my direction, I became frozen, penetrated painfully. I knew he could not see me, even though he was inside of me. With the force of my entire will, I projected my consciousness deeper into his, until merely seeing would be superfluous: he could not help tasting me, feeling me, sensing me in every cell.

When I had his full attention, I communicated to him a passage I had read in the *Zohar* about soul mates:

"'And when the souls are created, male and female are within them together, as one. Later, when they descend to this world, they are separated from each other, the male from the female. The Holy One, blessed be He, reunites the separate male and female soul into one again. It is in their passion for each other that the two souls become one again.'"

He replied directly to my consciousness:

"'Happy is the man who through his deeds merits the chance to meet his soul mate. They will unite the male and the female, as they were before they came to this world.'"

"I'm glad you also study Kabbalah," I continued. "I have trouble with this logic."

I felt the warm glow of his amusement, "You cannot study Kabbalah; you must experience it."

"I don't understand."

"What does 'Zohar' mean? The 'Book of Splendor'—the splendor of full knowledge of God. Yet, there is no 'knowledge' of God, don't you see, because God is not a mental construct. Therein lies the paradox that creates true 'knowing' without the mind, or rather, that transcends the mind. The enormity of God must be sensed on all levels of your being, and to do that you must first embrace all aspects of your *self.* We are created in God's image, after all. He gave us a physical body, an energy or etheric body, an emotional body, a mental body, and a spirit body. All of these make up the consciousness—not just the mental body. You obviously *know* this. Why can't you *live* as if you do? 'Music, for me, has always been much more about, well, just doing it . . . about passion,' I believe you said. What kind of self-delusion is that? You are too disconnected from your body for that to be true. It is all about the mind for you: the need to understand in order to maintain control. Yet, Kabbalah is about understanding you can never understand. As soon as you *think* you have found the way, you are so lost. Get out of your head."

"I'm afraid."

"*You,* afraid? And a little while ago, you were accusing me of fearing your darkness—yes, I heard you. It goes both ways . . . let me teach you about darkness."

Clenching his fists, Paul raised his arms in the air like he was being crucified. As he did so, his form melted into a slightly younger version of himself: a mid-teenage Paul. Blood began to pour from the vertical scars along the veins in his wrists.

The room began to grow dark: I knew that I must return before losing consciousness. Still, I had one more question—an important one. I struggled to formulate the thought, to project my waning bit of energy: "But, I don't understand . . . if you've truly experienced God, how could you try to kill yourself—what kind of paradox is that?" My thoughts felt about as powerful as a key-chain flashlight in a fog. I could not wait for an answer: I was sinking fast. I needed a trigger phrase to anchor my consciousness, to get me back, to help me remember . . . *Zohar!* One word was all I needed. *Zohar. Zohar . . .* I repeated the trigger word over and over . . . and over and . . .

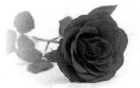

chapter 4: PAUL

February 1987
the same evening

Whatever made me think I could be a composer in the first place? Wherever my brain's been this evening, it certainly hasn't been on the music. Sometimes, it seems there is nothing more complex in the universe than putting notes on a page. Why did I sign myself up for this abuse? The irony is that I almost need to abuse myself in order to create. To live the abstraction that is music means disassociating myself. What did the poet, Arthur Rimbaud, call it?—*dérangement tous les sens* ("deranging all the senses"). Destruction to uncover creation. In the end, it's all about the body. "Yup, in the end, it's all about your dick!" That's what my old basketball coach used to say. Funny how true that ends up being—metaphorically at least. Even if you're not the kind of guy to give in to that, well, you spend a good deal of your energy—and therefore your attention—*not* giving in to it. How the hell did I get here anyway? Oh, now I remember: I was thinking about Dawn. I wish I didn't remember. It's bad enough that she keeps creeping into my mind every time I try to write. I have to forget about her. For one thing, she's too young. I don't want to hurt her. God, a sixteen-year-old girl's not even full grown—they look like they are; that's the problem—but they're not—inside. Besides, there is something not quite polished about her yet—not quite balanced. Well, she is young; time will take care of that but . . .

My head was swimming as I packed up my gear to head out for the night. *So long, studio 3—here's to a lot of wasted efforts!* I ripped up several sheets of erasure-stained manuscript paper and threw them into the trash. Well, on to the next mind-numbing endeavor: I was on my way to meet Gina.

As I made a left out the studio door, whom should I see sitting on a hallway bench but Dawn. She had manuscript paper strewn from end to end, hogging the entire seat like a child's train tracks across a living room rug. She looked ill. All of a sudden, her pencil fell to the floor. She looked confused, staring at her hand as though it were a foreign object. Then, she looked up and gave me a weak but surprised smile: "Oh, hi."

"Hi, yourself." I picked up the pencil and handed it to her. "What are you doing here?"

She smiled again, nodding toward the pencil. "Uh . . . my roommate has company," she replied, "and all I need is a little corner in which to work. I have to complete this flute sonata for Amy Hagaman by tomorrow. She's going to premier it at her recital at the Second Presbyterian."

"Why don't you just use a studio?"

"I like the hustle and bustle out here: it's a bird's-eye view. I can feed off the collective energy. Besides, I would feel guilty taking up studio space, since it's so competitive—and I don't need a piano to compose."

Damn, I thought. "Well, you certainly have been keeping busy," I offered. "I just saw a flier announcing your recital at the Museum of Art . . . and another one at the United Methodist Church."

"Yes, and did your buddy Kevin tell you that I'm writing a trumpet concerto for him?"

"No, he didn't," I responded with genuine surprise. "But I thought you were concentrating on performing." I then raised my voice about an octave to imitate Dawn's: "'There will be time later to compose, to be intellectually fecund.'"

She was not amused: "Why must you constantly throw my words back at me?"

"Constantly? I don't recall having done that before."

"Oh . . . whatever . . . anyway, I *am* concentrating on performing. This year's *Concours Reine Elisabeth* is for piano, and I'm applying. That is, I *have* applied . . . mostly."

"Mostly?" I tried not to reveal in my tone how impressed I was. The Queen Elisabeth of Belgium International Music Competition was huge in the classical music world. Even competitors who placed low in the standings would brag about being good enough to apply.

"I sent in my application materials—minus the requested letter of recommendation from my major teacher. I knew it'd be difficult to obtain one from Professor Fichet, since he doesn't show me much support. I half-hoped that they would overlook it, once they saw my performance credentials. Well, they didn't; I received a letter from them more than a week ago stating that the recommendation from him is mandatory. Since then, I've been trying to get Fichet—the butthead—to write one for me. He's been dragging his feet. They gave me a deadline of next week. . . . I really want to do this." Her voice had a frenetic tone.

"You want to do a lot," I stated flatly.

"Well, as Segovia said, we have 'an eternity to rest.'"

"Hah! You think we rest in eternity?"

"Uh," she stammered, "I guess so, in a manner of speaking . . . at least we find some sort of peace."

"Maybe we only have peace if we deserve it."

"What do you mean?"

"Maybe we have to come back until we get it right."

"Ah, reincarnation." Something in her eyes began to grow cold. "I'm surprised you believe in that, being Jewish like me."

"Actually, I don't. It does go against Jewish sensibilities."

I was surprised to find out that she was Jewish because she looked so Japanese with her almond eyes, straight black hair, high cheekbones, and tiny features. The only incongruous attribute was the blueness of her eyes, which I had presumed—based on her last name—came from some German ancestor. To discover that she was German-*Jewish*, like myself, was a pleasant surprise. I wanted to ask her about this, but the heat of debate had already inflamed my ego.

"There is nothing mutually exclusive about Judaism and reincarnation," she began off-handedly. "In fact, the early Hebrews embraced reincarnation as an accepted belief. There is evidence that the earliest scriptural writings contained passages concerning reincarnation which were later removed to distinguish Judaism from other faiths."

"That may be, but modern Judaism certainly does not support a belief in reincarnation," I asserted.

"Nor does it support disbelief," she quickly countered. "The Ashkenazim—from which most of us Jews in America have descended—were far more into practices than theology. As such, modern American Judaism is very practical, focusing on what we can *do* today, leaving what we may or may not *know* in the hands of God. If you think about it, that kinda leaves the door wide open— metaphysically, so to speak." She smiled with self-satisfaction. As annoying as her intellectual hubris was, it was damned cute. Nonetheless, I could not let her off the hook too easily.

"Although it is true that the Talmud never addresses what happens to the soul after death, I think this is due more to the rabbinical belief that such discussion is idolatrous than to an atti- tude of 'anything goes as long as you observe the Sabbath and don't eat pork.' Many rabbis still see transmigration of the soul as an affront to monotheism," I contended.

"Of course, as you said," Dawn replied gently, "we are cre- ated in God's image . . ."

"When did I say that? I don't remember saying that."

"Oh, I guess I must have misunderstood you," she said quickly, rubbing her forehead in defeat or just plain weariness. Either way, I felt for her, and my tone became more gentle: "You should get some rest."

Again, the weak smile. "Haven't you heard the nickname I've been given around here?" she asked with rhetorical cheeki- ness. "They call me 'kinetic' because I'm always in motion—a blur of creative energy. A body in motion remains in motion and all that. I can't stop . . . or I'll crash. You probably wouldn't know anything about that—you're so staid and composed. You proba- bly don't know anything about uncontrollable hyperactivity. I'll bet—"

"Hold on," I interjected. "When I was seven, I was too hyper to attend my own birthday party! I bounced off the walls—literally. We had this couch in the den, and I would run down the stairs, leap above the couch so my feet tapped the wall behind, and spring onto the couch like a Slinky. I was always getting into trouble for my ups—and later, my downs—until . . ."

"Until what?" she asked gently.

I heaved a big sigh and went for it: "Until they learned I was manic-depressive." There. I said it.

"Oh. Is that all?"

"Is that *all?*" I was confused by her nonchalance: was it courage—or ignorance?

"I just mean you're in good company . . . so was Tchaikovsky . . . and probably Rachmaninov . . . and countless other great writers, thinkers, and painters. Although hardly a prerequisite for artistic greatness, it's certainly not a hindrance."

Okay; so it wasn't ignorance.

"Now I understand why you're so staid," she continued. "Lithium, right?"

"Something like that."

"Is that why you tried to kill yourself?"

"How did you know that?" I asked nervously, wracking my brain for a way she could.

"The scars on your wrists."

Oh. I thought my penchant for long-sleeved shirts pretty well took care of that. I guess I was wrong.

"It's okay—you don't have to talk about it," she said quickly, apparently interpreting my thoughtful silence as avoidance. Perhaps she was right. "Maybe you should pray to your ancestors for guidance," she deadpanned.

"Excuse me?" I chuckled.

"No, I'm serious. My mother was raised as a Shinto-Buddhist, and she used to do that . . . quietly, of course: my father is Jewish, and the household has always been Jewish. In fact, my mother converted to Judaism, but she used to have this unobtrusive shrine that housed a bunch of little dolls. Sometimes, she would take out the dolls and kneel before them. Once, I asked her to explain it to me, and she just told me that the dolls represented our ancestors and that she was praying to them for guidance."

"Do you believe the dolls were your ancestors?"

"I said they *represented* our ancestors . . . Anyway, I believe the dead are energy, which is available to us—if we are open to it."

"What happened to the shrine?"

"I don't know. Maybe my father burned it."

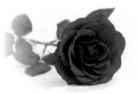

chapter 5: DAWN

May 1987

Edwin Eisenbach, M.D., OB/GYN. The name was emblazoned on the otherwise stark door in big gold letters. It made me think of the movie, *The Ten Commandments,* when the fiery finger of God inscribed Moses' tablets with the Law. I wondered what fervent hand had given this man so much authority. Well, the nurse at Peabody said he was the best . . .

"Insurance card, please," the receptionist said crisply as she pulled back the glass pane and held out her pudgy little hand.

"I—don't have one."

The receptionist's nose suddenly seemed quite a bit longer as she glared down its full length in an attempt to make me feel small—as if I didn't already feel bad enough. I was practically ready to puke at the prospect of what lay ahead.

"Well, you'll have to pay the full cost of the office visit, then," she said coldly. "That will be one hundred, payable by cash or check. We don't accept credit cards—or deferred payments."

I swear she added in that last remark just for fun.

"I can't pay one hundred dollars today."

"Then you can't see the doctor today—it's as simple as that."

Okay, she really was getting way too much enjoyment out of my embarrassment. I'd fix her fat ass.

"Oh, I'm so sorry. Now I remember," I replied, summoning up my sweetest voice. "I *do* have my checkbook with me." I dug to the bottom of my large purse and pulled out some checks from an account I had closed two months ago. Thank God, I never threw anything away. My mother had always nagged me about pack ratting. *See, Ma—I knew it'd pay off someday!* I wasn't particularly worried about what would happen when they found out my check was no good; I'd talk my way out of that like I had talked my way out of so many things before. At least this transgression would get me in the door today.

"Here you go, ma'am. I'm sorry about the confusion—just having a slow day," I purred while handing over my hot check.

"That's okay, I understand," the receptionist mimicked my tone in bewilderment. "You may have a seat." She actually looked like I had just slapped her.

The waiting room was packed with pregnant women, so I felt a little out of place. I had never been to a gynecologist before. I slumped into a corner chair as far away from the other women as possible. Based on my interchange with the receptionist—and my resale-shop clothing—they probably thought I was some kind of street urchin anyway. I picked up a six-month-old copy of *Parenting* magazine to thumb through because I liked the picture of the baby on the cover. He had a big hopeful smile on his face, and his arms were reaching eagerly above his head in an effort to be picked up. I had always loved babies. From the outset, it seemed I was destined to be a mother.

When I was a little girl, my favorite toy was a baby doll that I really loved. I used to hug her, kiss her on the face, and dress her every day, rotating her outfits as though she were a real child. My mother even sewed a coat and hat for her. I named her Bayou after the song, "Blue Bayou." I didn't know what the song meant, but I thought Bayou was the most beautiful name ever. It seemed to suit my baby girl—indeed, she had blue eyes.

For my fifth birthday, someone gave me a toy baby carriage as a present, and then there was no stopping me. I wheeled Bayou around the neighborhood like the proud parent I was. Many of the little boys would stop their games of dodge ball or tag to investigate my baby coach. Sometimes, they would look inside; sometimes, they would just follow me, inquisitively, from a distance. A curious foreshadowing of adulthood, now that I think about it. I was irresistibly drawn to the doll, or more specifically, to what the doll represented—a baby—without understanding why. In the same way, the boys were irresistibly drawn to me *with* the doll, or what this represented—motherhood—without knowing why. My maternal vibrations pulled the boys into my circle of influence like a queen bee attracts her drones. The biological pull sure begins early.

Another time, several of my boy cousins were visiting, and one of them brought his favorite toy: a shiny new crawler crane. An odd specimen to me, girl that I was, with its geometric design and pointy ends. It was like the big men, with their square bodies and angular minds. Still, there was something endearing about this object, cute in a way that a boy is cute—in his straightforward design. It was a strange comfort, coming from the complexity of softness that is girlhood, and I wanted to embrace this manifestation of maleness in the only way I knew how: as a female. I took the crane gently in my tiny hands and placed it alongside my doll baby in the carriage. I put a blanket over the two of them—the doll baby and the crawler crane—to show them equal regard and tenderness . . . like any good mother would.

Yes, I loved babies.

Yet, the reason I was at the gynecologist's office today had nothing to do with babies—it had to do with pain. For the past few months, I had been having terrible pain—the kind that wakes you up at night and haunts you during the day, gnawing at your patience, your self-image, your hope. It was there all of the time—a grinding ache that always seemed busy; however, it was much worse during my period, when it felt like I was being split open, eaten alive, from the inside out by some cannibalistic monster. The pain was so bad I could not remember the physical sensation of it—my mind blocked that out. Only the intellectual knowledge that it had been unbearable remained. Also, about two months ago I had started to experience bleeding that was not my period. The first time this happened frightened me, for the blood was very different from menstrual blood, which is thick and plushy with uterine tissue. This blood was thin and bright red—like the blood from a knife wound. It was as if I had been shattered deep inside, and tiny slivers of my self were cutting inward.

"Miss Wassmer, my name is Pamela, and I'll be your nurse. Please come with me."

I followed the round, middle-aged blonde through a heavy swinging door to a narrow hallway, which flowed directly into a rather large examining room.

"Take off all your clothes, including your underwear," ordered Pamela. "You can use one of the gowns—opening in the *front,* please—that you'll find in the drawer to your left."

I waited for a moment to see if Pamela would leave, but she remained, flipping furiously through the many papers on her clipboard. I sighed and slipped off my Docksider loafers while unbuttoning my blue blouse. Slowly, I removed my plaid skirt, folding it carefully to protect the pleats, and laid it gingerly against the back of a chair. Pamela glared at me with a look of impatience, so I picked up the pace, stripping to my bra and panties.

"Remove *all* your clothing, dear."

"Uh . . . there are no gowns in here," I said nervously, leaning on the drawer handle for support, totally in the nude.

"That's all right," Pamela chirped. "I'll find you one momentarily, but first we must check our weight."

I couldn't help smiling at that. I had a pretty good idea of what Pamela weighed: too much. With my arms across my breasts, I walked timidly to the scale, keeping my back to her as much as possible.

"You're in a doctor's office, dear," she purred as condescendingly as an alpha Siamese. "There's no need to feel embarrassed."

Excuse me if I feel embarrassed stepping on a platform in my bare ass.

"Oh my," she breathed, clicking her tongue. "Eighty-nine pounds. You are a thin one, aren't you? Have you been screened for an eating disorder?"

"Yes, about once a day—by *somebody's* grandmother."

"And you're an uppity one, aren't you?"

"Yes, that's right."

"Well, Miss Uppity, the doctor will be in to see you shortly."

"What? I don't have to enumerate all my symptoms for you, only to reiterate them when the doctor appears?"

"That won't be necessary," Pamela said dryly. "The questionnaire you filled out will suffice." She started out the door.

"Please don't forget my gown," I called after her. "I don't feel like playing Lady Godiva today!" Why was I being so incorrigible? It must be fear. Whenever I became frightened, the snippy little brat in me came alive. There didn't seem to be much I could do to hinder her awakening.

I removed my blouse from the chair and put it on so that the buttons were in back. This way, my front would be covered. Sitting on the examining table with my legs dangling off the side, I suddenly felt very small. To my right was a table containing myriad scary-looking instruments worthy of Dr. Frankenstein. There were claws and blades, circles and sticks, long skinny metal objects that seemed to make no sense: scissors without sharp edges, screwdrivers without heads. Would any of those go inside of me? The mere possibility made me cross my legs.

On the far wall hung a print of a painting by Edouard-Bernard Debat-Ponsan, which I recalled from my Art History class was entitled *Motherhood*. It depicted a peasant woman happily carrying her baby girl along a dirt road, accompanied by a cow and her calf. For me, the juxtaposition of the two families—human and bovine—made a statement about acceptance. The natural order was to have babies, and to therefore be tied to the biological urge to have babies. It was natural and right, and we shouldn't question it.

On the adjacent wall was a print of Picasso's *Maternity*. The angular face of the nursing mother looked a little too serious as her eerily thin hands enveloped her tiny baby, of which only a profile of the head and one miniature hand was visible. The baby's hand rested on Mama's bare breast.

I found these images of woman's reproductive responsibility to be quite droll, given the surroundings. Glancing back at the table of instruments, I thought: *All this for freakin' babies?* Wait, how could I think that? . . . Fear was definitely in the driver's seat.

If I had to choose a painting for this wall, it would be Marc Chagall's *Pregnant Woman Maternity.* A faceless woman with a see-through belly, standing on unsteady ground. *That's* how I felt: exposed yet invisible.

The pain had certainly made me feel exposed about a week ago. I had been arguing with Paul when it seized me . . .

"You would say that about any girl who wasn't you!"

His words shot through me like a vaccine. They were in response to my frustration at his still seeing Gina.

"But I don't understand," I said with strained voice, fighting back the tears. "We have the same mind, the same heart. How can you even spend time with someone else? How can you bear to be with her if you care about me?"

"I care about you, that's true—but such a relationship between us is impossible. I could never think of you in that way. Look, wouldn't it be nice to have that other person—that romantic interest—independent of what we have? What we have is so cerebral, so spiritual. Why taint it?"

"How can love taint anything?"

"Because with love comes all the ugliness: jealousy, fear, pain, uncertainty, longing, the need to possess, to control. None of that is necessary with a spiritual union."

I decided to take a different approach: "But Gina is abrasive and manipulative; you've said so yourself."

"Well, yes . . . but she's cute."

"So. There are many cute girls who aren't abrasive—or manipulative."

He smiled knowingly. "Like you?"

"I didn't say that. Look, for a person like you, Gina could be very destructive: she knows what she wants, and she has no compunction about taking it. As for you, well, let's just say, you go with the flow, allowing others to—"

Paul interrupted: "You mean I have no direction and can be easily led!"

"I didn't say that, come on . . . what I am saying is this: you are by nature self-destructive and are therefore attracted to dangerous people like Gina. Subconsciously you know this—that's why you find her attractive. However, consciously, you simply find her fascinating."

"As I said, you would say that about any girl who wasn't you . . . hey, what's wrong?"

"I—don't know," I gasped through clenched teeth. "It—just hurts. It isn't the first time." I bit my lip.

"Have you seen a doctor?" Paul asked, looking concerned. "You're awfully pale."

"No, I . . . I'm not sure whom to see."

"Well, at least talk to the nurse. She would know whether you're in any imminent danger. You honestly don't look very well . . . you really need to see the nurse." The worry in his voice intensified with each word.

It was nice to know he worried about me—nice to know he cared enough to give me advice. I had taken his advice; I had seen the school nurse. That is how I ended up here. . . .

"Hello, I'm Dr. Eisenbach."

I shook the large hand that was extended in front of me. "Pleased to meet you."

The doctor was an older man with gray generously splashed through his short, thinning brown hair. He had a wise, rabbinical look, due to his beard, wire-framed spectacles, and gentle brown eyes. Although he was not tall, he was a big man in terms of build: his large bones were well padded. I had hoped he would be a small man—that is, a man with small hands.

"Let's see," he began in a commanding voice. "You've been experiencing irregular bleeding and pain . . . can you describe the pain?"

"Yes: it hurts," I said wearily.

"Could you be more specific?"

"It's lower down, cuts deeply into my back, and it's sharp— jagged and jabbing. Sometimes, it takes my breath away; sometimes, it feels like it's squeezing—like I'm a wet towel, being wrung dry."

"Well, that's certainly descriptive."

I heard the snap of a rubber glove.

"How old are you, Dawn?" The doctor asked.

"Seventeen."

"Are you sexually active?"

"No—I'm a virgin."

"Good for you. . . . Pamela . . ." the doctor shifted as the nurse entered the room. "I think we'll need a smaller one of these." He held up a metal object that looked like pincers with a pointed beak.

"What is *that?*" I gasped.

The doctor smiled slightly. "It is called a *speculum.* It is used to hold the vaginal walls open so I can see the cervix."

Oh, goodie.

"And Pamela, could you bring this girl a gown?"

"Right away, Doctor," Pamela responded deferentially.

Had she simply forgotten—or was it some sort of pay back? Well, it didn't matter, for in a few minutes, I was in my gown— and the speculum was in the doctor's hand.

"Slide your bottom down here," he ordered, while motioning with his left hand. With his right hand, he snapped the stirrups from their dormant state, innocuously folded like wings against the body, into a more threatening stance. With the stirrups in the air, the examining table looked like a pterodactyl ready to attack. I placed my feet in the creature's claws . . .

I couldn't believe that asshole, Fichet: after saying he would write a letter of recommendation so I could attend the Queen Elisabeth *if* I altered my interpretation of the Tchaikovsky Piano Concerto no. 2 to be less—what did he say—*obscene,* he deliberately missed the deadline! And after I spent the whole winterim break on it, too! I swear that man is against me, and he's my major teacher—he's supposed to be *for* me. If only he had written that letter, I'd be in Brussels right now. The competition starts tomorrow—how's that for irony? The offer from that guy at the Künstler Höchster agency is looking better all the time. . . .

Oh, God! I feel like I'm being torn in half!

The doctor had just inserted the speculum in one forceful thrust and was opening the blades inside me. I heard the click, locking this intruder in place. My insides felt like they were burning and ripping at the same time. My legs began to shake: I had never before felt such invasive pain. Involuntary tears began to fall.

I could see a giant cotton swab entering my vagina; it was accompanied by deep, edgy cramping. The speculum was then removed, only to be replaced by two brusque, indifferent fingers. I felt a sudden sharp pain at the center of my being as the fingers moved. The other enormous hand began prodding my abdomen.

"Tell me if I touch anything that hurts," he said, suddenly making me recall there was a person present.

"I—c-c-can't—tell," I choked.

There was simply too much pain to allow separation of one sensation from another, in the way that a depressed person cannot distinguish genuine tragedy from perceived insult.

He removed his hands, and the squeak of Latex rang in my ears like a liberty bell: my body was my own again. The white glove sailed into the trash.

"You can get dressed and meet me in the consultation room to the right," the doctor said curtly while exiting.

Pamela offered her assistance, but I shooed her away without speaking. I just wanted to be left alone. Impatiently hopping off the table was a mistake: my legs were shaking so much I nearly fell. My insides still burned and ached. I noticed that the tendrils of hair over my ears were wet. Somehow I managed to dress and make my way to the room next door. Feeling wobbly, I was relieved to sink into the comfortable chair that faced Dr. Eisenbach's desk.

"I really can't find anything physically wrong with you," the doctor began, his eyes not meeting mine.

"What do you mean *physically?*"

"I just mean that I see no signs of organic disease. You're certainly tender in some spots, but I think, primarily, you're just out of balance. At your age, we don't need to get too aggressive, so I think the best course of action would be to give Ortho-Novum 1/35 a try."

"You mean birth control pills?" I asked incredulously.

"Yes, that's right. It is the easiest—and the safest—way to regulate the menstrual cycle and reduce cramping. Besides, you'll probably be attending college soon. Am I right?"

"Actually, I am completing my sophomore year in college," I countered proudly.

"Really? At seventeen?" The corners of his mouth dropped in contemplation. "Well, that's all the more reason."

"I don't understand."

"Well . . . you're at a very fertile age. Oral contraceptives are simply the best way to go for a college girl. After all, you may want to become sexually active . . ."

"No, I *don't* want to," I said hotly.

Funny, I thought feminism was all about the freedom to choose.

"In any event," he sidestepped, looking amused, "try it for three months and see what happens." He took a prescription pad out of his pocket. "I'll write you a script. Come back in three months. See my receptionist on your way out for an appointment."

And that was that.

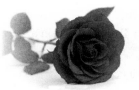

chapter 6: PAUL

January 1988

The disillusionment had been harsh and brutal, hacking through the delicate membranes she had so painfully grown to connect herself with him, leaving her with the shock and the torn bleeding ends of all her out-going feelings.
—Anna Kavan

The Peabody roof was a world unto itself—less so for the panoramic view of Baltimore than for the quick escape from the stresses of conservatory life. Although it was a forbidden area (a fact which, no doubt, increased the thrill), students continued to use the roof as a kind of sanctuary. Locks were picked, chains were cut, backs were watched—we all stuck together where the roof was concerned, even giving each other privacy when needed. To date, no student had fallen through to the floors below—despite warnings to the contrary.

Tonight was a good night for the roof: crisp and cold—perfect for clearing the mind. It reminded me of a certain night one year ago—*My God, had it been that long?*— walking home with . . .

Suddenly, Dawn appeared. Out of the shadows.

"How did you get past the guard?" I asked.

"I still have my student ID. I'm only on a leave of absence, you know."

"Does that mean you're coming back?"

"That's just one of the things I want to talk to you about."

Dawn and I had not talked in over two months, not since she had abruptly left school in mid-semester—though she had tried calling me recently, speaking only to Gina. Nonetheless, I had thought of her often. In fact, it was scary how much of my consciousness had been devoted to her. What had gotten in the way?

"I heard about your surgery," I said cautiously. "I was . . . worried about you."

"Evidently not enough to contact me," she snapped.

"I'm sorry about that, but . . . I did have my reasons."

"Evidently."

She stared at me for a moment, as if taking in the specimen before her. Then she blurted: "How could you have done it, Paul? How could you have moved in with her?"

"What I'd like to know is how the hell did you find out, anyway?" I countered, annoyed enough by her tone to match it.

"I called your parents," she smiled devilishly.

"In Seattle?"

"Yes, they weren't hard to find . . . that's how I got your new number. Your mother likes me."

I'm not surprised; the old bitch hates Gina.

"Yes, well, Gina doesn't—not anymore. She said you were faking your illness." *Now why did I tell her that?*

"Did she?" Dawn's eyes began to glare as her voice became louder. "Well, let me tell you just how much I've been faking! It has taken three doctors to find what's the matter with me. The first doctor, by the way, whom the school nurse recommended was an idiot." She paused to ensure her slur against my advice achieved full impact. "The second doctor was no better, but then I found a nice lady doctor who really knows her stuff. She examined me, realizing that the pain I felt *during* the exam was a definite sign. She simply said: 'I think you have endometriosis, but I can't be certain without a laparoscopy'—"

"Whoa," I interjected. "You'll need to define your terms."

"Well, okay. Endometriosis is a disease in which pieces of the endometrium—the tissue that lines the uterus—grow elsewhere in the body—usually on the ovaries or fallopian tubes, but sometimes, in the intestines, lungs . . . even the brain. Since this nomadic tissue responds to monthly hormonal fluctuations in the same way that the resident uterine tissue does, it bleeds—except there is no way for this blood to leave the body, causing internal bleeding, inflammation, and the formation of scar tissue. Eventually, adhesions bind the internal organs to one another. The pain is excruciating.

"The only way endometriosis can be diagnosed is with a laparoscopy, a procedure in which a small lighted tube—the *laparoscope*—is inserted into the navel so that the adhesions and scar tissue can actually be seen—"

"So, the doctor becomes kinda like a submarine captain, surveying the black oblivion through his periscope?" My attempt to lighten the mood.

Her eyes flashed in a moment of anger, but she continued, unabated: "First, however, the abdomen is distended with carbon dioxide to push the bowels out of the line of fire. This gas, by the way, doesn't leave the body right away; it lies in a pocket—around the breastbone and behind the shoulder blade—creating a sharp pain until it's ready to leave. And there's not a damn thing you can do about it."

"Sounds painful."

"It is! And you want to know the worst part? Before I went under, they only told me about the tiny incision in my navel. Then I woke up with *three* incisions—two of which are not so small!"

"Why three?"

"Well, one was for the actual surgery—the repair work, so to speak. I guess my growths were too extensive to just laser to death through the scope. I'm not entirely sure what the other incision was for—maybe some kind of clamp used to hold things in place—or move them out of the way." She shivered slightly. "Don't ask me; I was only the patient."

"So, they removed all these growths from your body?"

"Unfortunately, endometriosis doesn't work that way; it is akin to the beast, Hydra—if you destroy one of its heads, two grow in its place."

"So, what's the answer?"

"Well, there's this nasty drug, called danazol, that uses a synthetic male hormone to bring on pseudomenopause. It causes deepening of the voice and hair growth—not to mention the usual menopausal symptoms. By the way, it costs more than two hundred dollars a month! Since the birth control pill, with its pseudopregnancy state, has also proven to be effective by creating a much thinner than average endometrium—which carries over to the implants—I thought it would be worth a try. Besides, it's about one-tenth the cost of the danazol!"

"But what causes this problem in the first place?" I asked with genuine curiosity.

"They don't really know for sure, although there are several theories: immune problems, genetics, hormonal imbalance, retrograde bleeding. I even read somewhere that it is possible to be born with neutral cells that mutate into uterine lining when the hormones kick into high gear during puberty. Since this tissue is *outside* the uterus, its slough cannot leave the body in the normal manner. Consequently, it bleeds into itself."

"What is retrograde bleeding?" I asked.

"Well, during menstruation," she looked away as she said the word—girlishly silly, considering the nature of our conversation, "the fallopian tubes can carry uterine tissue back into the body."

"Ah, I see . . ." I had no idea what to say after that: I looked down at the floor.

"That's all you have to say?" she growled.

"What can I say? I'm sorry, of course . . . but what good does that do?"

She shrugged, stepping onto the ledge, looking down without flinching. "Gosh, I love the winter. The air molecules slow down when it freezes; they can't hold as many impurities." She inhaled deeply, and her body swayed.

"If you are trying to worry me, it's working."

"You do care about me—at least a little . . . I still can't get over Gina saying that I haven't really been sick!"

I should have known she would not let that one go. "I challenged her on that comment, believe me," I offered.

"You're pathetic, trying to play one woman against another—just like Dr. Zhivago." Dawn jumped off the ledge, and for a moment, all I could see moving toward me were two intense eyes.

"What the hell does that mean?"

"Guilt, rage, fear—whatever the motivating factor is, it's all about the man—his love of self . . . not of woman."

"Oh, that's rich! Are you telling me this entire conversation has not been about you?"

"That's just like a man, turning things around! The only reason you would even notice that is because it is so unusual for a woman's issues to be the center of conversation between a man and a woman. It's a sticking point in your head since it happens so infrequently—and you are so accustomed to being the center of attention . . . thank you for making my point for me!"

"How did this become a 'man vs. woman' thing? This is about you and me. Yes, I guess that's it, right there: is that why you sought me out—to argue, to attack me? I honestly don't understand what you're about . . ."

She gave me a look of disgust, then turned away. Silence. With her back toward me, she spoke quietly, deliberately: "You want to know what I'm 'about'? Okay, you asked for it. How many times have we talked about going to Europe? Hmm? Answer me."

"I don't know," I shrugged. "A lot, I guess."

"Precisely. So why are you going with her?" She turned to face me. "Yes, I know about your Fulbright grant application to study in Bern next year! I also know that Gina is studying there, too." I opened my mouth to speak, but Dawn held up her hand. "Before you ask, Kevin told me everything—we've become good friends since the première of my trumpet concerto, which, incidentally, garnered some recognition for his technical prowess. . . . I also recall that Gina's father is a real *gontser macher* in that international organization of music festivals, or something, the headquarters of which is also in Switzerland. I'll bet—"

"It doesn't work that way," I interrupted angrily.

"Don't tell me! I've been in this sleazy business all my life; I know exactly how it works—use and be used. You know how badly I wanted to leave last year, how unappreciated I am in this damned place! You said you had to stay, that everything you needed was here. You wouldn't run away with me, but you'll go to Bern with her? You stayed for *her,* but you wouldn't leave for me . . . and now, you're leaving with her?"

I could barely look at Dawn: her eyes were so sad.

"It's not the same," I tried. "You were asking me to throw everything away and bum around Europe with only the hope that we'd land somewhere useful. I am going to Bern specifically to earn a master's degree in composition. That's a big difference."

"You're still going with her and not me," she replied with an eerie flatness.

"Excuse me if I don't understand the urgency here. I'm not leaving for another eight months. . . ."

"But I'm leaving next week." Her words cut like ice in the cold night. All I could do was stare. "I've signed with the Künstler Höchster agency in Vienna—a two-year contract," she continued. "I'm going on tour. They've been hot on my trail since the Yale Gordon. Anyway, I need the money . . . having to leave school due to illness left me with a pile of bills and a transcript of Incompletes. Theoretically, Peabody reimburses you for the time you do not attend; however, after they nickel and dime you and apply their quirky percentages—well, let's just say there is not much left—certainly not enough to make a dent in the following semester's tuition. My father's struggle with cancer has kept him out of work for over a year, so I can't afford to return to school."

"How can you leave your father?"

"He's actually doing better now. In fact, he has taken some contract work at Columbia Artists, which means he'll be staying in New York for a bit. I can't believe it: years of being an entertainment lawyer, working for artists; now, he's going to become a turncoat and work for the agents."

I smiled slightly. "That is interesting." I couldn't think of anything else to say, knowing how much she loved her father, knowing how puny the scholarship committee could be.

"Of course, there are many, many back bills to pay. . . ." Suddenly, Dawn grabbed my arm. "Why not come with me to Vienna? With your magnificent sense of orchestration, I'll bet you could find work conducting. With that, you could make the proper contacts to have your own works performed. Come on! What good are all these degrees except to teach? Is that what you really want to do—teach? Why not just *do?*" Her voice was as frenzied as a Tchaikovsky climax, which achieves full impact only through contrast with the enigmatic elegance that precedes it. Such impromptu passion was difficult to resist. Yet, resist it, I must—although why, I was no longer sure. I pulled away.

"You think you're so wise, so noble, so spiritual," she screeched, "but you're nothing but a selfish man. You only want to do the right thing, so you can feel superior, so no one will hate you!" She began to cry. "Well, I hate you. You've made me pathetic—"

"Don't say that," I blurted out in a pained voice.

"But it's *true,*" she sobbed. "Look, I'm begging you to be with me! How pathetic is that?"

"You are putting me in a bad position. I can't just kick Gina to the curb. What kind of person would that make me? You already accuse me of being selfish, but wouldn't that be the worst kind of selfish? I'm sorry if I led you on, but my initial attraction to you—on all levels—was so powerful I just couldn't ignore it. Yet, you must understand—I know you understand this—I'm committed to Gina. If I hurt her, I destroy who I am, everything I stand for, and I would be no good to you."

"What I cannot bear is that her potential pain is more important to you than my present pain."

"Why are you doing this to yourself?" I felt my exasperation mounting as I ran nervous fingers through my now moist hair. "You could do so much better than a struggling composer. Any available man would marry you. Why, I wouldn't be a bit surprised if you return from Vienna and introduce me to your husband."

Her eyes inflamed with increased rage. "You want me to find someone else! That way, you won't feel responsible—or guilty."

"Oh, whatever," I threw up my hands. "I can't talk to you when you're like this."

"Like what?"

"I don't know—goofy, irrational. How can such a brilliant woman be so stupid?"

"I'm not stupid . . . I'm just in love!"

Wow. This was the first time she'd said it.

"Don't you understand?" she continued tearfully. "You hurt me more than anyone I have ever known because I let you in more deeply. Like Dulcinea said to Don Quixote, 'Of all the cruel devils who badgered and battered me, you are the cruelest of all!'"

"Please, Dawn, please understand," I said slowly, painfully. "I have to stay: I'm graduating this year. I've worked so hard for this—harder than you've ever had to work." I was instantly sorry I had added that last bit; however, her mind could not be derailed. Lucky me.

"Don't try to distract me! I know what the real issue is: either you really love her—or you're the biggest chump in the world."

"Either way, I'm not worth losing any sleep over."

"Okay, okay. I'm a little dense sometimes, but I get it now." Her face assumed a look of resignation. "You don't want this to work. The trouble is, I've grown to need you."

"I need you, too."

"So, what are we going to do about that?"

"I don't know . . . stay in each other's lives . . . see what develops. Look, what do you want me to say? I do care about you." My gloved hand reached to wipe the moisture from her face. I couldn't tell if it were tears—or remnants of the snow that had begun to fall.

She turned away, but I could see her lips tighten, exposing teeth.

"Does it still hurt?" I asked.

"Yes, if you must know," she sighed, looking at me out of the corner of her eye. "More than I can bear sometimes."

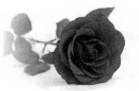

chapter 7: DAWN

March 1988

Wien, Wien, nur du allein—"Vienna, only you alone." Just like the song says: there is no city on earth that compares with Vienna, with its peculiar mix of old-world sensibilities and modern materialism; with its chocolate and cobblestones, tradition of excellence, and reverence for social grace. It is a city whose streets are safe enough for a woman to stroll alone at 2:00 a.m., and upon which the only women wearing pants are foreigners who don't know any better. It is a city where homelessness is not a civic concern—compassion for mediocrity is simply not allowed—where even waiters go to school to learn their trade, where no one is ever rushed out of a restaurant.

The image of Mozart—usually a stately silhouette of his profile—is everywhere: billboards, coffee cups, menus. Mozart. Irreverent composer who ended up in an unmarked pauper's grave, a fact which tour guides are quick to point out is no reflection on how Mozart was treated. "Mozart was highly respected in Vienna," they cluck proudly, while escorting both the artistically inquisitive and the historically dutiful through his former home at Domgasse, #5. A mere four years later found Mozart at the dismal Rauhensteingasse, a few hundred yards away in distance but miles away in prestige, slaving away on *The Magic Flute* and the *Requiem* with death—and his creditors— gnawing at his heels.

In addition to being the birthplace of a number of Mozart's masterpieces, including eleven piano concerti and *The Marriage of Figaro,* the Domgasse (literal translation: "cathedral lane," from its proximity to St. Stephen's) was also home to the first Viennese *Kaffeehaus,* in the seventeenth century.

The many faces of coffee in Vienna reflect its shades of contradiction. The vast gray area between black—*einen kleinen Mokka,* or "small strong black coffee"—and white—*eine Melange,* half coffee and half milk—makes having "just a cup of coffee" either a moment of festivity or confusion, depending on your point of view. There is *Kaffe mit Schlag*—coffee with cream; *einen Kapuziner*—with whipped cream; *einen Einspänner*—with whipped cream in a tall glass; *einen Türkischen*—prepared Turkish style, in a copper pot; and—the hallmark of Viennese sophistication—*einen Braunen*—with a splash of milk.

It is all about the experience, and nuance is clearly important, be it of manner, expression, or the experience itself. This is reflected in the language, for Viennese German is much more kaleidoscopic than the speech of the *Vaterland,* replete with gradations of formality and descriptive diminutives. For example, the Viennese fondly refer to the 448-foot-high steeple at the top of

St. Stephen's Cathedral as *alte Steffl*. Knowledge of German is not required to understand the cozy familiarity intended by this pet name. However, there is nothing diminutive about the cathedral, which is a sprawling hodgepodge of architectural styles from thirteenth-century Romanesque to fifteenth-century Gothic. Its asymmetry seems strangely endearing. In fact, its contradictions make it even more Viennese. All the streets of the *Innere Stadt,* or "inner city," seem to pull life from this enchanting ecclesia, despite its dark, mausolean form. The dark edges and angles are life-affirming in their defiance, in their refusal to be categorized. Austerity and ecstasy have coexisted here for centuries, steadfast through rampage like the Viennese spirit, itself.

The eclectic cathedral is a microcosm of the monumental Ringstrasse encircling the *Innere Stadt.* Here, instead of one building, there are seven (plus a few less-impressive landmarks), collectively creating a kind of exposition of European history in architecture. Conceived by Emperor Franz Josef in 1857 as a glorification of Vienna at the heart of the Austro-Hungarian Empire, the buildings serve as a flagship of the Modern Age.

The Parliament was built in Greek Revival style, while the *Rathaus* ("City Hall") is of Gothic design, as is the *Votivkirche* ("Votive Church"). The *Universität* (University of Vienna), the *Burgtheater* (National Theater), the *Naturhistorisches* (Museum of Natural History), and *Kunsthistorisches* (Museum of Art History) were built in the Renaissance Revival style in homage to the age of free thought. All the buildings symbolize periods of historical significance and, in turn, the boulevard is symbolic of Vienna itself, the quintessence of European culture, having sampled it all, savoring only the finest. Like the canvass of an Ayn Rand novel, the Ring—as it's fondly called—is a snapshot of humanity at its best, full of optimism and potential.

It was difficult to weigh such all-embracing liberalism against the myopic atrocities of the Nazi regime. How could I respect what the city represented and yet bury the knowledge of past horrors endured by my people? It was strange to be comfortable and yet on guard—strange to hide my Star of David inside my blouse, while saying *Gruß Gott* ("God's Greeting") to passersby, like I had lived here all my life.

I recalled that it had taken Leonard Bernstein—an American Jew—to give Mahler, an Austrian Jew, back to the Viennese. My father had shown me a video of Bernstein rehearsing with the Vienna Philharmonic, haranguing them in perfect German to embrace Mahler as *their* music, to take pride in it. Mahler was as Viennese as *Wienerschnitzel,* yet the Viennese had snubbed him for years, in the way that the German society had often condescended to anything that was not classified as Aryan. Mahler was one of them; his music was innately Viennese, yet they turned on him because he was a Jew—even though the vast majority of the Germanic intelligentsia were Jews.

What was it about this society that took credit for the best and blamed others for the worst? And yet, how does this differ from any other society known to man?

In the end, the Viennese people are no worse than any other—perhaps just easier to criticize because they are so privileged—but easier to respect because they have overcome so much misguidance and are still proud.

I was eighteen and had dreamed of Vienna all my life. I was not disappointed. What a glorious thing, to not be disappointed. It happens so rarely to those of us of high ambition, those of us who strive to succeed, achieve—even when we are not sure what it all means.

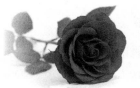

chapter 8

the pen is mightier than . . .
March 1988 through June 1988

Pension Aclon
Dorotheergasse 6
A-1010 Vienna, Austria
den 3. März 1988

16 E. Madison Street
Baltimore, MD 21202

Dear Paul,

Happy Birthday, you old man—twenty-four candles—oy, vay! I'll bet that cake looks pretty bright . . .
kinda like the Milky Way. I haven't heard from you, so
I decided to write again. Did you receive my last letter?
You can write back . . . I won't mind. Staying in touch
does require a joint effort (!)

I think of you often. What am I saying? I think of
you all the time: you're ingrained in my consciousness,
always there, as close as my own soul. I hate the way

we left things at our last meeting, but I was hurt. I'm still hurt. First of all, I don't understand: If you were so devoted to Gina, why did you approach me? How can you still be devoted to her if you love me? Perhaps you don't love me; perhaps you're only drawn to me intellectually. I keep rethinking what you said about friendship versus romantic involvement—how it would be nice to keep romantic interests separate so as not to taint a spiritual union. The more I think about this, the less sense it makes to me. How can a strong romantic relationship exist without the foundation of friendship? How can two people who are both relatively normal sexually not be romantically attracted to each other if there is a solid spiritual union? The only possibility would be that either one or both do not find the other physically attractive— even so, why would this be an impediment? I mean, how superficial does one have to be to sacrifice a spiritual connection for a predominately physical one?

Many times I have asked myself how you could be attracted to her and to me at the same time. Gina is . . . well, promiscuous, and I am not. I know guys often find promiscuity desirable, but I thought you were different. Maybe you're just ambivalent about your ideal woman: good girl versus bad girl. Maybe sexual experience doesn't—or shouldn't—make a girl "bad." Maybe I'm just an over-analytical pain in the ass.

Speaking of ambivalence, I must admit that it is strangely comforting to be removed from being so near and yet so far from you. At the conservatory, I could not bear to be away from you, nor could I bear to be in your company—unable to touch you, to possess you. Being in the same room, longing to speak of love and being only able to speak of the art we both shared, wrenched my soul. You would say it was impossible—this love between us. As much as I have tried to understand this, I cannot. Sometimes, I think I have figured it out, only to have my emotions take over, showing me a different reality. Then, I know that all my rationale was simply just that: rationale, with no basis of emotional or spiritual fact. Spiritual fact? Now, there's an oxymoron . . . or is it? I often sense in my soul—or feel in my heart—far greater truths than my mind can ever conceive. I sense that our meeting was no accident, that we were meant to connect, and that we will be connected forever in a way I don't fully understand.

There I go again: trying to understand. If only I could just feel without the need to analyze my feelings, perhaps, then, I could be happy. Perhaps, then, I could savor the half-cup that is mine, instead of spilling it upon my white dress while reaching for the whole cup I will never have. Yet I cannot turn off my mind; it sticks like a scratched record that can't sing past its scars, locked in a refrain of its own making. I still cannot understand why, if you were so intent on being the "good guy" and doing right by Gina, you approached me. Why did you express interest? Why did you offer me that reflection of my self in your eyes, only to pull the mirror away, leaving me trembling from withdrawal? The very thought of this renders me without thought. I am dumb; I am desperate. I am selfish and unworthy of your reply—and I hate you for making me unworthy.

Love,

Dawn

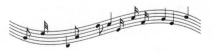

16 E. Madison Street
Baltimore, MD 21202
March 20, 1988

Pension Aclon
Dorotheergasse 6
A-1010 Vienna, Austria

Dearest Dawn,

After reading your letter, I had to put it aside for a few days because I was so angry. Rereading it, I just felt sad. First of all, you must understand, I met you at a time when I felt lost within my ideals—alone and misunderstood. Your soul is my soul, so it seemed as impossible to turn away from you as to cut out my own awareness. You and I have both been warped by life: bitterly disappointed with people, dimmed by struggle. The only difference is that you still want to fight back. You cannot accept the possibility of a purposeless cycle—I can. I don't have the need to change the world. Every action we take does not have to be one of courage, one of daring. Sometimes, the unchampioned responsibility taken with no expectations is heroic enough.

You ask: "How can a strong romantic relationship exist without the foundation of friendship?" Well, sometimes a romantic commitment occurs before there is time to determine whether or not an underlying friendship exists. What does a decent person do in this situation—just spit in the face of the attentions this other person has shown him? There is also the possibility that, while in this relationship, not having experienced anything better, he could presume that there is nothing better— only to be proven wrong by meeting someone else. Then, what does said decent person do: trade in what he has for the new-and-improved model?

You also ask: "How superficial does one have to be to sacrifice a spiritual connection for a predominately physical one?" This is not even relevant, for upon finding themselves in a "predominately physical" relationship, most people are quite surprised to be there and, in fact, only discover their predicament by comparison with some very different relationship that has just happened to come along. By then, of course, it is simply too late—if one has any conscience at all.

"How can two people who are both relatively normal sexually not be romantically attracted to each other if there is a solid spiritual union?" Well, perhaps they are—but that does not mean they have to act upon it.

What else can I say? I do love you, and I want to be your friend. Why can't that be enough?

Love,

Paul

Pension Aclon

Dorotheergasse 6

A-1010 Vienna, Austria

den 3. April 1988

16 E. Madison Street

Baltimore, MD 21202

Dear Paul,

I'm feeling desperate; I can't think; I am so unworthy. Whenever I see happy couples, I hate them. Why do they deserve such fortune, while I do not? Why must I love someone whom God has not given me? Why must my life be nothing but struggle and work? It is difficult to remember why I am working so hard. Is it simply to forget all the horrible, miserable, lousy feelings? I am so broken inside. Sometimes, I can't believe how much. I don't understand why it hurts so much. The only way to stop the hurting is to stop being myself. As soon as I reconnect with my identity, the pain is right there to greet me.

I want to look in your eyes, to hear your breath. Do you miss my physical presence at all? Do you ache to be near me? You say you love me. You could not be so matter-of-fact if that were true. You would do whatever it takes to be with me. Love is willing to go to Hell to be with that person, to face destruction for passion's sake, to risk everything for a single kiss—like Dante's Francesca and Paolo, doomed to the second circle of the *Inferno* for succumbing to that kiss of "wholly trembling mouth." All the rest is just talk.

Vienna is full of lovers—and children. When I see them, I scream inside. The lovers make me feel inadequate; the children just make me sad. I remember too well what it was like to be so vulnerable, to have such high hopes. They are so fragile, it makes me cry. They desperately seek approval. They love their grandparents, who are also fragile. A small group of students has sought out my services as a result of a series of church recitals I have given. One of the little girls I teach was so excited because her grandparents came to visit. She wanted them to sit in during our lesson. I allowed it because of my memories of what it was like to have grandparents, to want to impress them. I want to feel deeply again in a good way. And yet, the melancholy has always been part of my being. I am not sure it was ever absent—even in the face of joy. "There is no greater sadness than to recall a happy time at a time of misery," wrote Dante. Well, I think it is even sadder to recall a happy time and realize that, even then, the misery was still there. What is wrong with me? I feel everything so deeply that the most mundane event can crush me into shards. I just want to be like everyone else—but if that is not possible, I want to learn how to excel. If I must suffer, let me at least be great. How do I get there from here? And if I stop to love you, will I ever get there? But how do I go on without you? The future without you seems so bleak, I almost don't care what happens. I think the emptiness wherein lies the facing of oneself is the most frightening place in the world. Without you, I will be forced to go there. Does that make sense? I don't want to hide behind my love for you, and yet, being in your presence makes me content. Contentment breeds mediocrity, I know that—but does that mean to be great forces one into an eternal state of discontent? What a trade-off!

I have been dabbling with drinking to ease my pain. Wine and beer are so abundant here—and so acceptable. I had my first shot of brandy a few weeks ago. I never felt anything like it. The liquor massaged my brain until all the anxiety turned warm and fuzzy. The problems were still there, but somehow I seemed to be facing them with a clearer head, like my mind had just gone white-water rafting and returned refreshed. Since then, I have experimented with a couple of shots, which usually leave me sprawled on the floor, unable to stand. It's a nice feeling when the anguish is severe. It is light and airy—transcendent. Dare I say, it is the closest experience on the physical plane to my spiritual journeys—and the side effects are no worse (!)

My concert in Budapest last week was a smashing hit. The Hungarians love me! I think it might be because they, too, do not shy away from suffering, trying to be gracious in the face of it. They do not storm their obstacles; instead, they devise clever ways around them—even dishonest ways. There is an often misunderstood courage in this, I think.

I played the Prokofiev Two. The guest conductor, Esa-Pekka

Salonen (you know, the principal conductor of the Swedish Radio Symphony), had requested the Prokofiev Three, but I am saving that one. It is my fantasy to play this concerto with you conducting. How's that for choosing "our song"?

Vienna is still a city of music and musicians, but it is also a fantastic base of operations because of its proximity to all the great cities I want to conquer. Budapest, Bratislava, Prague—even Berlin and Dresden—are accessible by train. Speaking of which, I am leaving for Germany tomorrow, where I will be playing in a total of six cities. Then, I'm on to Poland to play with the Wroclaw Chamber Orchestra. So, if I don't write for a while, that's why.

Love,
Dawn

Pension Aclon
Dorotheergasse 6
A-1010 Vienna, Austria
den 5. Mai 1988

16 E. Madison Street
Baltimore, MD 21202

Dear Paul,

Okay, just because I was on the road, does that mean I didn't deserve at least one measly little note? You know, you're really hard on my insecurity. Sometimes, I wish I had never met you.

Poland was creepy. The agency screwed up my visa—the one I was issued allowed me to visit, but not to work—so I was detained in a Wroclaw jail overnight until they straightened the whole thing out. That was scary: there I was, not speaking a word of Polish, in the hands of communist officials. Not an experience I wish to relive. Needless to say, I was relieved to return to Vienna. It is strange how comfortable I have become here. My one redeeming memory of Poland will always be: after my concert, a communist, atheist woman gave me a hug and announced: "Now, I understand God." I can imagine no greater compliment.

Love,

Dawn

16 E. Madison Street
Baltimore, MD 21202
May 18, 1988

Pension Aclon
Dorotheergasse 6
A-1010 Vienna, Austria

Dear Dawn,

Your letters have given me much to consider, and my delay in responding has been because I didn't want to make matters worse. I wanted to be certain that my own confusion did not hurt you more. I am torn between doing the right thing by Gina and my love for you. I know you have a difficult time understanding this, but it is the way I feel. What you said that night on the roof of the Peabody . . . about Gina's father helping me to study in Switzerland . . . well, you were right. So, you see, I feel a certain loyalty to her. What kind of person would I be if I didn't? More to the point, if that were the case, why would you want me?

Frankly, I was also damned mad at you for doubting my feelings.

How could you question my love for you after all we have communicated to each other? How does a commitment made prior to meeting you detract from this love? Your insecurity concerns me, and I suspect it is not entirely—or even primarily—my fault. In fact, I am fairly certain that the real reason you feel so despondent has very little to do with me. Forgive me if I sound like a psychologist, but years of being psyched out myself must have rubbed off; so, I'll continue this logic and ask you about the source of your insecurity. Do you know? Do you have any idea why such a talented and beautiful woman would doubt her power over men enough to waste her energy worrying about whether or not I'm available?

 With love,
 Paul

16 E. Madison Street
Baltimore, MD 21202
June 2, 1988

Pension Aclon
Dorotheergasse 6
A-1010 Vienna, Austria

Dear Dawn,
 So, now *you're* the one who doesn't write back! Did my last letter scare you? I hope to hear from you soon. By the way, I'm a college graduate! It is difficult to believe I made it. Playing by the rules does have its perks. *Répondez tout de suite, s'il vous plaît.* I'm worried about you.
 Love,
 Paul

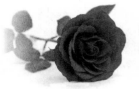

chapter 9: DAWN

August 1988

I sat at the Café Central, wishing I had a big, fat American bagel to go with such a divine cup of coffee. Talk about irony. The bagel has become so ingrained in American culture that few realize it was actually founded in Vienna, originally baked as a symbol of military triumph. After King Sobieski of Poland led his cavalry to victory against the second Turkish siege of Vienna in 1683, the round pastry supposedly shaped like a stirrup—*Bügel* in German—was created in his honor. Despite the power of this image, the bagel no longer graced the shelves of the Viennese bakery. The irony was taken one step further by the fact that the best cream cheese I had ever eaten had been in Vienna: *Liptauer*—paprika cream cheese—and *Kräuter Gervais*—cream cheese with chives. Both were richly creamed but with a tangy bite.

Well, even if they did serve bagels here, I probably couldn't afford them. The Café Central had been, in its heyday—before the world wars—one of the most famous cafés in Europe. Perhaps Leon Trotsky and Stalin had played chess at the very table where I sat. Many famous artists and writers had practically lived at the Central, since extremely overcrowded apartment houses had been the norm, due to Vienna's population surge. At that time, apartment space had been sublet literally by the square foot, and people of limited means had often been able to afford just enough to house a single bed. I smiled to myself as I thought of so many of my contemporaries, living in spacious homes yet seeking out cafés in which to create because they deemed it romantic or inspiring or whatever, when the real reason artists began working in cafés was because their actual living spaces were untenable.

Struggling to find work in the wasteland that is the European music scene in summer, bouncing from cheap to even cheaper rooming house, I was as close to this artistic ideology as I wanted to ever be. Believe me, it was not romantic. It was degrading, exhausting—even terrifying at times—but definitely not romantic. Perhaps, however, romance only exists in retrospect.

Because of its illustrious past, the Central's menu was rather pricey, particularly for an out-of-work musician. Yet, coffee was such a way of life in this city that one could linger for hours—no matter how crowded the establishment—over a single cup of coffee, thereby softening the sting of the investment.

Funny how coffee came to Vienna around the same time as the bagel: during the same Turkish siege, the victors found sacks of brown beans abandoned at the sultan's army camps.

As it turned out, Franz George Kolschitzky, a well-traveled merchant who had been spying for the Viennese, had sampled the dark brew, known as *Kahve,* in Turkey. Quick to seize an opportunity, he opened Vienna's first *Kaffeehaus,* and coffee became ensconced in the culture. Meanwhile, the bagel never gained a foothold. It only goes to show how difficult it is to predict what will catch on . . . and to think that I have based my whole life's work on the unquantifiable whim of human taste.

And yet, I sought comfort in my belief that there is always some logic—no matter how distorted—in what rises to the top. As I sipped my *Melange,* I realized that, of all the coffee creations, this enticing synergy of half coffee, half steamed milk best summed up the undercurrent of the city: deep, dark bitterness smoothed with creamy whiteness to make it easier on the stomach.

Perhaps this was a skill to be learned from these crafty Viennese. I, with my prickly directness, could use some of that. How, for example, could I smooth over the bitterness of my past—and even my present—to make it more palatable to Paul? I hadn't written him since May because things had become difficult after that. Work had dried up, and the agency had not returned my calls. I had been homeless for a time, bouncing around with different folks. How could I tell Paul that? What would he think of me . . . particularly since it had not been the first time? How could I tell him that, before we met, I had lived with three different women, that I had run away from home at age fourteen, that when I had applied to Peabody, I hadn't even a high school diploma, that Peabody had offered me only a $1,000 scholarship out of $7,850 tuition, that I had been homeless before, that . . .

I noticed that a Pomeranian was licking my hand. The experience gave me a glimpse of home, for in Vienna, dogs were taught to observe the barriers of personal space almost as well as their owners. As I turned my American-trained palm to envelop its tiny head, I thought about trust. This dog's skull could be crushed by my hand, made powerful through years of scales and arpeggios. Yet, he just sat there without fear, lovingly licking my fingers. I sensed the intensity from his little body: he knew compassion, forgiveness—trust. I did not feel worthy of him; I pulled my hand away.

All I ever wanted, as a child, was for my mother to look at me the way she often looked at my sister: with pride, entrusting all her dreams. I recalled my first juried exam on the piano. At the time, my sister and I both took lessons, so we were both participants. I received a glowing critique, and I ran excitedly to show my mother. She barely said a word. A few hours later, my sister emerged with a report that was nothing special. I could see the glow in my mother's eyes while my sister recounted every detail of her examination. My mother was completely transfixed, and I knew at that moment that no matter what I accomplished during my lifetime, I could never divert that glow in my direction . . . never bask in even a speck of it.

My parents bought their first piano so my sister could play. They dreamed of turning her into a great virtuoso. She progressed slowly, however, and when I, toddling along behind, quickly outshone her—accidentally, spontaneously—no one was happy. Frequently while practicing, I would be assailed by my sister that I was "hogging her piano," even though she hardly ever practiced herself. Rather than defending my dedication, my mother finally demanded I leave the piano to my sister, with the words: "We bought it for *her,* anyway!" Events such as this may seem small, but I have met folks in their seventies and eighties who still recalled similar cruelties from childhood with a look of pain. It is scary what shapes us, humbles us with the fear of flying. This fear is often ingrained by those above whom it is our greatest wish to soar, while they, from the ground, regard us in awe.

Paul had asked me to reveal the source of my insecurity to him. Although initially I had resented the request, I was now glad he had made it, for he had forced me to look at my own scars. The only trouble was, I did not know how to communicate what I had learned to him. In the art of human relations, I still had a long way to go.

For one thing, my jealousy needed to be brought under control. It drained me, distracted me, kept me from being truly great. Yet, like a whirring air conditioner that grates on your nerves until you find that the sticky silence is even worse, I could not turn it off. As if my struggles to find work, friends, and even food were not bad enough, I continuously upped my misery factor by comparing myself to other people. Every time I thought about Paul, I became consumed with jealousy, obsessed with trying to figure out what Gina had that I did not. A family with money, for one thing, and connections. Yet if Paul were so superficial that he would be swayed by things like that, he certainly wasn't worth all this anguish. Could it be that all his pleas of loyalty and "doing the right thing" were true? I couldn't understand that because, if a person's heart is truly with someone else, then where's the loyalty? In my mind, this would be even worse because on top of splitting his attentions, he would also be lying about it—to himself and to Gina. Wouldn't his so-called loyalty to Gina, in that case, be little more than condescension? And if all this were not the case, he was lying to me as well as to her. So, at best, he was a self-deluding, self-centered ass with an ego the size of Rubenesque hips; at worst, he was playing us both. Either way, he was simply not worth it, but still . . .

As painful as it was, I had never felt as intensely as I did where Paul was concerned, never felt so alive—not even for music. This frightened me, but enticed me, like the suicide that fascinates you even as you cringe "but for the grace of God go I."

Not only did I compare myself to Gina, but I compared myself to Paul. My insecurity could not allow me to be happy for him. When I thought of his bachelor's degree from Peabody, I felt a funny feeling in my stomach. His assimilation into conventional expectations made me feel the lesser somehow, as if his light could actually detract from my own brightness. I often doubted my choices, which created even more frustration because, in the final analysis, I felt I really didn't have a choice. Life seemed to yank and twist like Dali on speed, leaving me so accustomed to pain that the only thing I could do was blame myself for the things I could not change. It was a ritual that left me strangely satisfied.

I wish I could change Paul's do-everything-by-the-book attitude. He was so irritating, and yet . . . so cute. I swear, I didn't know where to land—kind of like the Viennese cream cheese with no bagel to be spread upon, nowhere to extend myself, no reason to make myself smooth.

That's it! I needed to find the reason, needed to smooth out the edges for my own sake. I wouldn't contact Paul again until I had done just that. He wouldn't find me attractive if he felt sorry for me; he couldn't know that I had fallen upon hard times or that I was mired in lovesick jealousy. He already knew far too much. If I proceeded along the same course, all the mystery would be gone, and he would lose interest for sure. But wait! He would be leaving for Bern in the next couple of weeks. How would I ever find him if we lost touch?

I settled myself with the thought that I could always contact his parents. They had been gracious to me in the past, so there was no reason . . .

So, it was all settled: I would find work—and myself—before I found him. And not before.

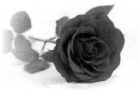

chapter 10: PAUL

September 1988

I can't believe I'm actually going to Bern to study with Theo Hirsbrunner, one of the few living composers I admire . . . probably the *only* one I admire! He, in turn, actually studied with Pierre Boulez—the greatest living tonal serialist. What did I do to deserve this? It is gratifying to know that my work is appreciated on some level, really gratifying . . . Wow!

Searching the corner of Gina's and my small apartment that I partitioned off for a studio—using a maimed cardboard box—I furiously try to figure out what books I need to pack. Maybe I should ship them. Maybe I should buy one of those fancy trunks. I suddenly realize that I haven't eaten anything today, but I don't need to eat: too full of energy as it is. "Fit as a fiddle and ready to go," I begin to sing, recalling the prosaic little melody from my old piano exercise books, *A Dozen a Day.* To conclude each dozen of finger exercises, there was a variation on the refrain, "Fit as a fiddle." Each set became increasingly difficult until they just positively blew your mind.

I want to be sure I bring plenty of my music, so Hirsbrunner won't think I'm a one-hit wonder. He really loved my piano concerto . . . everybody loves that damned piano concerto. Well, I'm damned sick of it. I've moved beyond it. Why can't they see that? I swear, they want to hold me back. I was hoping to complete that brass quintet before our flight and the song cycle on Whitman poetry and . . . where did I put those pens? *(Crash!)* Oh, I guess I yanked on that desk drawer a bit too hard. Oh, please! Now, I'll have to clean up all this stuff!

A strip of paper catches my eye: a fortune from one of those cookies at Uncle Lee's on South Street where Dawn and I once ate Sichuan. It reads: "Depart not from the path which fate has assigned you." Dawn. Where are you?

Peeking her head around the partition, Gina speaks: "Paul, did you take your lithium?"

Now, what is she trying to say? She knows I stopped taking it. I don't answer.

"Paul, you know you can't just stop."

"I can't compose when I'm on that stuff. It takes away my ups and downs."

"Well, yeah . . . that's kinda the point." She sighs wearily as she moves the box to give herself more room. She grabs my arm. "You can't work this way, either; you're spinning out of control."

So, now *she* is jealous, too? "What do you know? Is it control to do whatever you want and still feel nothing? That's how you are because you can *afford* to be that way. You play like you're hot, but it costs you nothing because you're really cold. The hair that falls on a barbershop floor has more feeling than you! What do you know?"

Gina's eyes flare, but her voice remains calm: "I know that whatever you write in this state ends up being garbage."

"Once again, how would you know? The only taste you have is in your mouth!"

She throws up her hands. "Look, the one thing I do know is that if you don't call Dr. Hutchinson, I will."

"Yeah, well, fine! If you think you're woman enough to gang up on me with Dr. Hutchinson, go ahead! But you gotta catch me first . . . I don't need either one of you. I'm a genius, do you understand? I don't need anyone's permission to exist; I just *am*. Screw you! I'm getting out of here."

"Where in the hell are you going?" Gina's face was blank.

"To buy a freakin' trunk!"

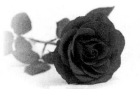

chapter 11: DAWN

November 1988

"Messages swarmed in my dreams in the night"
—As said by Solveig in Henrik Ibsen's *Peer Gynt*

The stairs of the Baroque town house, leading up to the tiny room I was lucky enough to afford, seemed to grow steeper and steeper. I felt dizzy, and my back ached. Sitting upon the step to catch my equilibrium, I leaned forward and pulled my knees to my chest for security. I could feel a tug in my abdomen, which was swollen and sore. The act of resting my breasts against my knees was painful, and in my legs, there was a strange tingling pain that I had never felt before. The step was wide and curved like a mother's lap, just not as soft, but I nestled against it as though it were and bit my lip as the tears began to fall. What was I doing here anyway, in this cold, aloof city where barely anyone knew me? Vienna was beautiful on the surface— serene and polished, enviably integrated. Problem was, it was *too* integrated. The society was so seamless, it was difficult for an outsider to snip his or her way in—particularly if one happened to be *her.*

If I weren't a woman, the Künstler Höchster agency would never have treated me so badly. Flashbacks of contract negotiations reminded me how much this was true. Caveats, clauses, and contingencies had been wielded against me like switchblades in a dark Baltimore alley, and as in that scenario, I had been simply grateful to escape with my self intact. Coming out on top had simply not been an issue. My questions and concerns had not been addressed, and I would have figured this happened to everyone, except for the fact that my rep had been abruptly called out of the office, giving me a chance to eavesdrop. The same rep had been speaking to another artist—a male artist—but with a completely different tone of voice. He had been patient, gracious, and accommodating, providing room for both elaborate questions and ample responses, even offering information beyond the request.

That had only been the beginning. In fact, this very morning, a more pertinent—and disturbing—encounter occurred. I had a meeting with Karl, the vice president, in an attempt to sell myself into better jobs. The meeting was going badly, and in defeat, I rose to leave. As I approached the door, Karl grabbed my arm, spinning me toward him. He unzipped his pants, then encircled the wrist of my free hand with his stubby fingers, yanking it until my palm fell on the head of his erect penis. The sticky wetness seemed to burn into my flesh. I tried to escape, but I could not. His face was so close to mine I could feel his hot breath. "There is an easy way to earn better jobs," he breathed. "Just be a good little girl and be nice to me." He tugged harder. "Come on, suck me! Put that little tongue of yours to work . . . then we can *both* have what we want."

As shaky as I felt, my voice remained firm: "Not on your life." I punctuated this with a look of disgust, which earned me a merciless shove, throwing me to my knees.

"Then get out of here, you useless idiot," he barked.

I didn't wait to be told a second time. The last thing I heard as I made my escape was: "You'll never work in this city again!"

The funny thing was, during the meeting, I had noticed a fax from the Vienna Symphony, lying on Karl's desk. They had to find a piano soloist, able to play Rachmaninov's Piano Concerto no. 2 with Leonard Bernstein the following night, since the scheduled artist had suddenly taken ill.

I immediately raced over to the symphony's administrative offices, hitting door buzzers at random until someone beeped me in. I stormed into the director's office, résumé and tape in hand, and demanded he give me a chance. The poor guy was flabbergasted. Business is simply not conducted this way in Vienna. Layers of ceremony and status that have taken generations to build cannot be sliced through with one stroke. The famed Vienna Philharmonic has never even had a woman in its orchestra, and I could count on one hand the number of female soloists that I could recall—mostly vocalists. Ah yes, the old "issue of blood" phobia: women are "unstable" and cannot be relied upon to put professional responsibilities first, due to hormonal fluctuations. The irony was that I actually played *better* when I had my period. My awareness—and therefore, my precision—was heightened.

Of course, such discrimination had deep roots among my own people in the belief that a woman was somehow "unclean" at this time of her cycle. I could never understand this. Hadn't the God we were supposedly respecting by keeping ourselves hidden created this process in the first place? When I was a girl, the Jewish faith, with all its colorful rituals, was beautiful to me—

grounding even. As I became a woman, I could not live with the contradiction of submitting to rituals that betrayed the very nature of my womanness. After all, God had created me, too.

Nonetheless, in Vienna discrimination was certainly not unilateral. Even a man had to be of proper lineage. Of course, the Vienna *Symphony* was not quite so elitist, but still . . .

I don't know whether it was due to shock or amusement, but the director *did* give me a chance: "I am afraid the final decision rests with Herr Bernstein, *gnädige Frau,*" he said softly. "He is staying at the Imperial."

That was all I needed. I made my way to the Hotel Imperial in record time. Unfortunately, the desk clerk was not so kind, and I could not wrestle Bernstein's room number out of him. Exasperated, I sat in one of the big, plushy chairs in the lobby, across from an antique grandfather clock, which kept perfect time. The lobby of this hotel was positively regal. From where I sat, I could see three chandeliers, ornate mirrors, and marble columns, leading to a breathtaking marble staircase. I had heard that guests could actually request how hard or soft they wanted their mattresses to be. Despite the pleasant surroundings, the loudness of the clock was irritating to my overwrought nervous system, yet I couldn't bring myself to move. I had played for Bernstein at Tanglewood when I was only ten, and he had been kind to me. I felt that we had a special bond, since he had given Mahler back to Vienna, and Mahler was an ancestor of mine. I knew if I could just get to him, the gig would be mine. But how? I closed my eyes and focused on the ticking of the clock, trying to tune into my surroundings, to become at peace with them— and with myself. I timed my breaths with every other tick: slowly in, slowly out. Then, I prayed.

The minute I opened my eyes, my body once again became rigid—but this time, with excitement. Whom should I see, exiting the hotel café? None other than Leonard Bernstein! He was with two other men. I tried not to think as I hurried toward them, my legs turning to jelly.

"Sir, my name is Dawn Wassmer, and I'm a pianist with Künstler Höchster. You and I worked together at Tanglewood nearly a decade ago. You said of my playing, 'She plays with more veracity than any young pianist I have ever heard.'"

The maestro stopped walking long enough to give me the once-over. A sudden look of amusement came over his face. "Were you even potty-trained a decade ago?" The two other men laughed.

"I was ten, sir," I replied without averting my gaze. "I'm eighteen, now. You said I had a promising future."

"Well, was I right? Is your present everything that your past promised?"

"I'm working on it; in fact, that is what I wanted to talk to you about."

I told him the whole story—even the part in Karl's office. I was amazed at my own words; I was even more amazed that he listened to them.

Nervously playing with his cigarette, as if unsure whether to smoke it or throw it away, the maestro seemed much older than he had eight years ago. I knew that he had celebrated his seventieth birthday a few months earlier. Nonetheless, he was still handsome and unbelievably charismatic. This maneuver had been worth it just to be in his presence—even if nothing else came of it.

During our conversation, he alternated between walking and pausing to look at me. I stayed with him, following him outside the hotel and into the street. The two other men had already gone their separate ways. Suddenly, we stopped. I noticed that we were at the Musikverein. Certain that I would soon be dismissed, I pulled out the big gun: "Mr. Bernstein, please give me this opportunity. I promise you will not regret it. Remember November 14, 1943 . . . remember when you stepped in for Bruno Walter at Carnegie Hall on a few hours notice . . . remember that after that concert—that opportunity—offers from all over the world began pouring in . . ."

He looked at me intently for a few moments that seemed much longer. I would have been frightened, except that he was so gracious, and in his eyes I saw only gentleness. Finally he spoke: "My dear young friend, since we're here anyway, I might as well have a listen."

And as they say, the rest is history. I still couldn't figure out how it had all transpired, even though the performance was tomorrow night. If only I didn't feel so lousy. All my confidence and spirit had been depleted obtaining this job. Now, what would I use to play it? Resentment filled my soul for all those artists who made it look so easy. It was not easy for me; it was killing me— yet, I could not live without it. My headache made it difficult to think sequentially. I felt like an open wound: painfully exposed, vulnerable to infection, permeable to touch. I didn't want to talk to anyone, yet I was afraid to be alone, afraid of my own dark thoughts. Gina and Paul. It hurt so much that my insides ached. Why couldn't I just forget him? Somehow, I made it upstairs and into bed without bothering to remove my clothes.

Late the next morning, I awakened in a pool of blood. How could this happen to me on the day of my most important gig ever, playing the Rachmaninov Second at the Musikverein with Leonard Bernstein and the Vienna Symphony? How could I be that unlucky? Ever since Tanglewood, I had dreamed of soloing with a major symphony under the baton of Leonard Bernstein. Jack of all trades, master of all, he was my idol. Everything he touched—piano, conducting, composition, writing—became magical. He was what I wanted to become. . . . Well, I should have known that my period was on its way from my twisted thinking, but there had never been any rhythm to my cycles except for those months I'd been on the Pill. Since I'd stopped taking it, my so-called cycles had become even goofier. . . . Besides, it was nearly impossible to perceive my distorted logic when I was in the middle of it—kinda like trying to fathom the full impact of a typhoon while being crushed between two waves.

Speaking of waves, the pain was surging and dissipating, contracting and releasing like a giant hand inside my belly. Soon the pain would be constant, and I would have no respite. There was always a narrow window between the onset and the apex of pain. I was grateful for this time to settle myself in a safe place before the monster seized the reins.

Now, I had to zone into crisis mode, to think like a warrior going into battle, which I was. Focusing the mind on the task at hand, one step at a time: that was the way to maintain control. What did I need to do right now? Stay ahead of this pain. I searched my room for wine, brandy—anything to numb my awareness. There was nothing. *Okay, that means I need to find something . . . quickly!* I thought. But first, I would have to clean up. Grabbing all the personal items my cloudy brain could register and praying that no one would see me in the hallway, I proceeded to the shared bath. . . .

My walk down Herrengasse became surreal. The pain was intense now, and my vision was narrowing, turning black around the edges. This cropped view gave me an artist's discernment into the underlying nature of things. The buildings breathed into the streets whose dinginess enveloped me like a dirty but familiar blanket. For a split second, I felt the pulse of creation—ecstatic agony—and I was not afraid. I channeled myself into the sidewalk and stone, into the energy bodies of passersby, into historic homes where the living and the so-called dead cohabited. As in Scott Mutter's *Surrational Images,* boundaries became meaningless. Townhouses bled; cathedrals glared with human eyes, shining with fluorescent light. Both man and the man-made seemed equally alive.

On the corner, I could see Vienna's first skyscraper, *Hochhaus,* or "high house," reflecting man's need to invade the sky, to reach for his creator. From this, I devised a koan: why does man use material to escape the material?

Why, indeed, as I sought to ingest a material substance to escape my visceral pain? For some reason, I could not find a bottle shoppe, even though I was certain there were several in this neighborhood. I approached Herrengasse 13—the *Landhaus*—where, on March 13, 1848, imperial troops opened fire on a crowd of demonstrators, killing five people. The revolution that followed was futile, the lives lost were wasted lives, little more than filler copy on the pages of history. Nonetheless, at that moment, their blood loss connected to my blood loss, and I could feel their wounds as my own, stretching across those questionable concepts of time and space. "One of those moments," as Anna Kavan wrote, "which seem to generate a sense of life's futility and sadness." Yet there was beauty in this connected sadness, strung across the city of man like Christmas lights that, even in their festivity, evoke a tugging sense of regret. . . .

The pain impaled me: a giant, jagged stake piercing through my lower back to my front or my front to my lower back—I couldn't tell which and didn't care—radiating down my thighs to my knees.

I always felt so powerless during the week before my period. Water retention altered the way I looked and the way I felt inside my swollen brain. (I had read that when a woman's ankles, fingers, abdomen, and breasts retain fluid, her brain does, too. This stretches the surrounding membrane until its sensitive nerves are shoved against the skull, causing dizziness, headaches, agitation, and depression.)

The only way to climb out of this black hole was to bleed— and for me, this meant experiencing extreme pain.

The male benchmark—to "push on," to assail your attacker—can never work in a woman's body. A woman's threats are internal, not external like, for example, war. If she rails against her threats, she is fighting herself. If she pushes onward, in denial, pain will force her to pay attention to her body. I was learning this.

I was learning that I could not deny the physical without losing the concrete reality of my intellect. Without the physical, the intellect is no better than a symphony that stays in the head, unheard except by its composer. I was learning how much men and women need each other—how much we have to teach each other . . . if only the male society could respect my female need to go into darkness . . . if only I could express the wisdom of this. . . .

I could no longer think or stand; I needed things to be simple. So, I went into the Café Central and ordered a glass of *Grüner Veltliner.* The unseasoned edginess of the local white wine suited my mood. My swallows were quick and deep. The potion found its way to my pain, working its magic like a masseur's skilled fingers.

Suddenly, I noticed a woman two tables away. She reminded me of Solveig, the woman who had helped me after I'd first run away from my father's house, the woman I had loved. Like Solveig, this woman was tall and blonde—the direct opposite of me. She had beautiful eyes—more intense than Solveig's and bluer. I hadn't known that was possible, but . . .

Wait; is she checking me out? Our eyes meet, and I look away—only to quickly sneak another look. *She probably thinks I'm flirting . . . am I? . . .*

She rose, moving toward me. Her movements were catlike. As nonchalantly as I could, I glanced upward to meet her eyes.

Me: *"Bitte, nehmen Sie Platz."* ("Please sit down.")

Her: *"Ah, Sie sind nicht Österreicherin!"* ("You are not Austrian!")

Me: *"Nein. Wohnen Sie hier?"* ("No. Do you live here?")

Her: *"Ja . . . jetzt."* ("Yes . . . now.")

Me: *"Woher sind Sie?"* ("Where are you from?")

Her: *"Ost-Berlin . . . und . . . Sie sind Amerikanerin."* ("East Berlin . . . and . . . you are American.")

Me: "Yes, I'm American. Please, sit down."

Her: *"Störe ich Sie?"* ("Am I disturbing you?")

Me: *"Nein, bedienen Sie sich."* ("No, help yourself.")

She took a seat, crossing her long legs. She was wearing a short skirt. "I'm Nadja," she purred with outstretched hand.

I took her hand and held it for a moment, trying to get a sense of the woman in front of me. She was strong and determined but not hard: firm grip but smooth, feminine skin. Not particularly pretty except for her eyes, she possessed that poised attractiveness derived from self-assurance, that sense of "I'm just fine by myself," which ironically compels others to "wanna play, too."

"And you are . . . ?" She added finally. I had forgotten to tell her my name.

"Dawn," I offered, my eyes focusing on her legs, very little of which were concealed by her skirt. It was a great skirt: blue, woolen, plaid. She also wore a black turtleneck, a blue scarf, and a long black cashmere coat that had seen better days. The dark colors made her blonde hair, which was in a chignon, glisten boldly like the sunrise rising from a dark night.

"*Ich möchte eine Melange,*" Nadja requested from the waiter in her crisp Berliner German, replete with the guttural *kh*. My father was born in Berlin, so the German I spoke was more like hers than that of the Viennese. This made us both outsiders.

I ordered another *Grüner,* as my pain, although somewhat numbed, was still sharp. Nadja commented on my periodic wincing, which I, at first, dismissed as "female trouble." Eventually, I told her the whole story. She nodded knowingly. "I had terrible pain all through my teens," she told me. "I lost four days every month. As soon as the pain began, I went into hiding."

"What did you do?" I took another swig of wine.

She smiled with embarrassment. "How do you say, 'the Pill'—it gave life back to me. Pretty funny . . . *me* on birth control . . . considering I don't like men. After a few months on the Pill, I said to myself: 'So, these are what they call cramps; I can live with this'—nothing like that horrible animal pain!"

"Animal pain. That's a good way of describing it." I offered a half smile. "I wish the Pill had helped me. Well, I guess it did— a little . . . but not enough to justify the headaches, nausea, and fatigue it caused. Plus, I didn't like being chained to this unnatural thing."

"Hah! *Was ist* unnatural? If humanity has access to it, then it is natural! 'Earth's crammed with Heaven, and every common bush afire with God.' That was written in your language." Nadja punctuated the *your* with a jerk of her index finger.

"Yes, I know—by Elizabeth Barrett Browning. One of my favorites."

"Ah, you like poetry!" She seemed inordinately happy with this discovery. As if sensing my perplexity, she offered: "I'm a poet myself."

"No kidding! A real poet, like with books out and all!"

Nadja laughed. "*Ja*, 'a real poet,' as you say, 'with books' . . ."

"Wow. If you don't mind my asking, how did a poet get out of East Berlin?"

Her eyes darkened. "*Das ist* . . . long and painful story."

Unpleasant subjects. We talked no more about them. Instead, we drank wine and coffee and ate *Topfenknödel*— dumplings with cream cheese.

"*Was für ein schönes Mädchen!*" ("What a beautiful girl!") Nadja murmured, while lightly stroking the outside of her fingers against my face. "*Und so schöne Augen* . . ." ("And such beautiful eyes . . .")

"*Ich bin nicht ein Mädchen.*" ("I am not a girl.") I countered. "*Ich bin fast neunzehn!*" ("I am almost nineteen!")

"I am not telling *my* age!" Nadja exclaimed. If I had to guess, I would have said thirty-five. "Listen," she continued. "I would like to show you my place. It is not far . . . I have wine there. . . ."

As we turned down the *Tiefer Graben,* home to some of the finest shops in Vienna, Nadja pulled a tissue from her pocket to blow her nose. She then flung it upon the ground with a flourish: "See, I'm an American, too!"

So, it's always there . . . almost as bad as being a Jew . . .

We veered onto a side street, where the shops were more individual and less pricey. A small apartment above an antique clock shop, Nadja called home.

As we entered, a particularly harsh streak of sunlight pierced through the dome light, further distorting my already distorted vision. *All the better to see you with, my dear!*

"The wine is in here," Nadja said as we approached the kitchen. "I have vodka, too—if you want. I'm half-Russian, so I always have vodka in the *Haus.*"

"Wine will be fine," I managed before sucking in my breath. The roaches were too numerous to count, moving faster than any creatures I had ever seen. They seemed highly positioned above the countertop, stilted on their skinny little legs. My sunspotted eyeballs saw them as rapid sparks, like the scene in the movie, *The Ten Commandments,* when Egypt was plagued by the hail that turned to fire. That movie had clearly made an impact on me.

Nadja snickered at my reaction as she poured some wine for me and some vodka for herself: "Welcome to the real world."

We took our drinks into the living room and, although there were several chairs and even a couch, sat on the floor. I curled into a ball against the pain.

"Let me try to help." Nadja's strong fingers began massaging the cords of tension that ran along both sides of my neck. As my neck softened, she followed the path of unexplored tension to my shoulders, which she kneaded like a French pastry chef: sensuously and skillfully. In her touch were power and gentleness, mastery and fear, light and dark. In her touch was . . . everything.

By holding my awareness to the prison of my body, Nadja was offering the key to its release. But the liberation was not empowering: my insides ached and quivered with fear.

Reaching my lower back, she recoiled suddenly, frantically shaking her hands.

"What is it?" I asked, almost with dread.

"The pain in your body; it's incredible. It is filling up my hands; I must shake it out. Your aura is so full of pain—I've never felt anything like it."

Well, I didn't know about my aura, but my lower back was certainly full of pain—so much that it was sensitive to the touch. The idea that her touch could be sensitive to the pain filled me with eeriness, suggesting more belief than disbelief.

By now, I was fully uncoiled from my fetal position, allowing Nadja access to my front. She began by stroking the center of my neck, then—gingerly—my breastbone. Her hand subtly but curiously slid beneath my sweater, brushing against my Star of David. She made a small noise but spoke no words as her fingers—now more gentle than strong—circled the nipple of my left breast, moving in such slow motion, they gave the illusion of traveling a great distance, of prolonging an already long journey. I felt an ache in my abdomen that was quite different from the one that had already been there. This one was pulling without being painful, warm and comfortingly familiar—even though I had never felt it before, at least that I could remember and certainly, not like this.

There had been this neighborhood boy who had tried to feel me up once, sliding his hand down my sweater, but it had hurt, and I had stopped him.

My thoughts turned to Solveig, who had saved me. Like an apparition conjured from the dew of dreams, that beautiful creature had stepped into my life at just the right moment. There had been nowhere to go, no one to believe in, and I had been so tired, so sick . . .

For a time, I even believed that I had dreamed her into my life, had drawn her to me by the hunger of my soul. Solveig. So aptly named. "Who would have thought I could draw you here / the way that I've longed to, by night and by day." They could have been mine—those words said by Ibsen's Peer Gynt to his Solveig. And I had failed my benevolent Solveig just as Peer had—by my own lack of courage, by the fear that my faith had instilled.

I thought faith was supposed to make you strong. It had not been that simple; it was never that simple. Why was everything so gray? I needed things to be either black or white, hot or cold. "Because you are lukewarm, I will spew you from my mouth." What did that mean? Perhaps it meant that to live as you truly are—no matter how contrary—is less sinful than living a lie.

My life with Solveig had been a lie. I hadn't meant it to be; I had simply been incapable of acting out my love. And Solveig would not just take that love, would not allow me such a convenient loophole. She had been older and had known better. "You're too young to understand what you want, too righteous to accept the consequences," she had said. "But I'll tell you one thing, if I were a man, I'd take you to that bed right now and fuck your brains out." Not being a man, she had never done any more than kiss me on the lips. . . .

I suddenly became aware of my wandering mind, which had been a defense mechanism against all those sensations I wasn't supposed to be enjoying. If I didn't respond to them, they didn't exist—and I certainly wasn't to blame. . . .

As hard as I tried, I could not block out these feelings that both frightened and delighted me. How could something feel so right and yet so very, very wrong? I was attracted to Nadja, but I knew I shouldn't be. I had been taught that to love another woman was an "abomination." And I could not turn off those voices any more than I could tune out my feelings.

As Nadja began to move her mouth toward my breast, I felt my body stiffen. She must have felt it, too, for she abruptly pulled her face away and began to remove her hand, brushing once more against my Star. This time, however, she seized the pendant, fondling its edges as though they were curves.

"*Ach!* You are Jewish!"

"Is that a problem?"

Nadja laughed sardonically. "Not at all. I am Jewish, too . . . that is, *Messianic* Jewish."

"Messianic?"

She gave me the same sweet smile one gives a four-year-old. "Messianics embrace the tenets of Judaism—except for one thing: we believe that the Messiah has already come. He is Yeshua, or, as you say, 'Jesus.'"

I had never heard anything like this before.

"Isn't that a contradiction in terms?" I asked, unable to conceal my confusion.

"Why?" Nadja shot back, her eyes probing. "The only reason Gentiles were allowed to receive the grace of the Messiah was because we Jews rejected him. He came for *us,* to fulfill the prophecy. 'A shoot springs from the stock of Jesse . . . he is the spirit of Yahweh . . . a spirit of wisdom and insight, a spirit of compassion and power . . . the spirit of Yahweh is his breath.'" She struggled to formulate her words, finally grabbing the Bible that was nestled, almost protectively, against the couch. She found the passage quickly and her face shone with peace while she read quietly to herself. Soon, the peace turned to anguish, and she shook her head, her eyes meeting mine in dismay and helplessness. "I am trying, but I can't translate it to English. You read German, *nicht wahr?*"

"Slowly." I took the book from her hands, noticing that it was opened to Isaiah, chapter 11. I had read this many times, but I couldn't recall having read it in German. The text seemed to speak differently to me this time, as I noticed allusions to Bethlehem and the line of David. *The wolf lives with the lamb, the panther lies down with the kid, calf and cub feed together with a little child to lead them* . . . I thought of Jesus and his championing of the weak, the humble; his willingness to throw the prescribed order off its axis for compassion's sake. I felt peace at these images, but also fear—almost as much as I had of Nadja. Was I having a spiritual insight, or was this simply a surreal mental state induced by wine, rapid blood loss, and heightened sexuality? Perhaps it was just the experience of slowing down my mind to read a passage I thought was so automatic in a language that was not, forcing me to look at every word. Perhaps this was just the key. Perhaps . . .

My old mind fought back: "What about 'I am the first and I am the last, and there is no God besides Me'? Aren't we challenging monotheism?"

Nadja smiled peacefully, knowingly, as though she were completely prepared for this. "Have you ever wondered why all the Hebrew words for God are in the plural: *Adoshem, Adonai, Elohim?* Doesn't that suggest to you that God is more than one aspect? If He created all things, how could He only be of one? *Der Vater und der Sohn und der heilig Geist.* Why would a human aspect of God suggest polytheism any more than 'man being created in God's image' would?"

I had no answer for that, so I decided to go for the jugular. "Okay, if you are so knowledgeable of the teachings, how do you justify loving other women?" I was immediately sorry after I had asked this, but Nadja did not seem to mind. Again, she seemed prepared.

"Of course, loving another woman is against the teachings. I know that—but so is sex of any kind outside marriage—so is even thinking about it, according to Yeshua's teachings. For that matter, so is thinking a single negative thought about anyone. Everyone's weakness—sin—is different. It is easy to judge a man who drinks too much and say 'he is going to Hell' if you can't even get the smell of alcohol past your lips. Being with you, like this, is my sin, and I know it. But it is *my* sin. What others find tempting—lying, stealing, killing—these have no hold on me. If I can go to God and say, 'Yes, I know I sinned with women, but it is my only uncleansed sin, and it was done out of love—not destruction. I loved the woman I was with; I cared for her and took responsibility.' If I say that, how can a God of love reject me? In any event, it is a chance I am willing to take; a chance I must take. There has been no place for me among men. Sometimes, it is not about what is 'right' but about what you can endure and still survive. Isn't choosing not to survive a sin, too?"

I did not answer, but I internalized her words. How was she any different from me, resenting the male society for not letting me retreat into darkness? My woman's spirit knew it could go anywhere, that the darkness was a necessary part of this freedom. My body, that had been taught to fight this darkness, was the only obstacle.

"'Sick with desire / and fastened to a dying animal / It knows not what it is,'" I whispered.

"Was?"

"Nothing, really—just a Yeats quote. I think it means that our death—and therefore our sin—often keeps us from knowing our true selves. The irony is, we long to connect the two: more than anything else, we want our despair to have meaning.

"Yet, God is outside any possibility of our knowing. Writing letters in the sky with our little-girl fingers—that is all of our theology. In the end, we pray to something that we have no idea of: faith is beyond everything and anything. You know what I loved best about Judaism as a child? The idea that God has no name— an inexpressible God. We cannot say his name because we are too small to encompass what we are addressing. When you attach a name to something, you put it in a box. It is the ultimate hubris to put God in a box. You must have the faith to pray into the vast- ness. The Western Wall is a great image—praying to a non- descript expanse that does not yield to our touch, our will."

I sighed and stood up, supporting my throbbing lower back with my hands. "Problem is, that is not enough for me anymore. I have realized that I don't know how to pray—at least, I can no longer feel it. I don't know what it all means."

Nadja, who had taken my cue to stand, walked over and put her arm around my shoulder. "Then, you must ask God how to pray. Even your confusion fits under God's vastness—the 'non- descript,' as you said. Sometimes, that confusion is all we have to remind us of our humanity—and our need of God. I think, our prayer life, if nothing else, is preparation for our relationship with God after death, so at least something in our moment of terror will be familiar. To accept that our most concrete relationship is not even concrete is our greatest obstacle."

"But sometimes it is difficult to find the strength when there is so much pain. It can all seem so futile," I wailed, surprised at my own words.

Nadja seemed suddenly exasperated. "Oh, here we go, the modern angst: life is futile, love is futile, having children is futile—*Scheiß*. Everything we do matters—even the most pathetic, jumbled prayer. This feeling that what we do is insignificant is just as much ego as thinking we have great impact. It is sheer ego implosion! Look at all the details of the world—the many species of birds and fish, the leaves on the trees. God is concerned with details, with small change. If He is not too great for this, why would we be?" She paused for a moment, then added softly: "And if he is not too big to concern himself with detail, why would he not deign to become human to save us?"

"Ah, what a surreptitious effort at conversion! I must admit, I have always liked the idea of God being born of woman, of God loving woman enough to come through her blood to reach man. When the girls in their Catholic school dresses spoke of this, I was always fascinated."

She leaned over as if to kiss my lips, but ended up kissing my forehead instead. "I wish men could realize how much *Mut* [courage] it takes to be gentle. Too many men feel they need to conquer to be strong. If anything, that just shows weakness and fear. Why can't they learn that there is nothing passive or banal about creation?"

She walked over to the window and stared upon the city, without words. It was an uncomfortable silence, but I dared not blemish it. I lay upon the couch as my body, once again, overtook me.

When she finally did speak, her words were far more disconcerting than the silence: "My beautiful city—when will it change?"

"What do you mean?"

"Destruction. It can happen quickly, when the need for conquest strikes—when armies swarm, devour—like those roaches in my kitchen."

"But they have done it before—it is still here . . . it *will* still be here."

"Not without much pain and suffering—and loss." Her voice suddenly sounded tearful.

"But that's what makes it beautiful."

I fell asleep then. It was a strange sleep: floating, dreamless, but somewhat conscious due to the pain. When I awakened, it was time to play my concert.

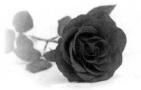

chapter 12: PAUL

November 1988
the same day

How the hell had I made it on time? Spending ten hours on the train, then going from bumpy train to buzzing *U-bahn* to pounding cobblestones had left me with a brutal headache. The pain radiated from the center of my forehead, forming an arch around my left eye. Could it be tension . . . or anticipation? Sometimes, a headache, for me, was a warning that my monster was about to strike. Trouble was, I never knew what side that two-faced sonofabitch was going to show.

I thought about Dawn and what she had revealed to me about her pain. I knew she suffered greatly, and I felt guilty complaining—even to myself. She made me want to be a better man, stronger for her. I just had to see her again . . .

I had lied to Gina, telling her that the agency with whom I had recently signed had offered me an impromptu gig as a stand-in conductor for the Budapest Radio Symphony. Instead, I had used my newfound contact—that Hirsbrunner had generously offered—to track Dawn's concerts. Evidently, he was a powerful contact, for he had heard early this morning about Dawn's last-minute booking with Bernstein and the Vienna Symphony. That had not given me much time to get from Bern to Vienna, but thanks to the high efficiency of the Eurail system, it had been possible.

The Musikverein was packed, and all three of its *Saals*—or halls—were in use. I made my way to the *Grosser Musikvereinssaal,* the largest of the three, where the symphony was already tuning up.

Built in 1869, the Musikverein was impressive, both visually and acoustically. The famed Vienna Philharmonic played here, as well as many other of the world's great orchestras while on tour. This evening, Dawn would be playing here with the Vienna Symphony, conducted by Leonard Bernstein. She would be playing the Rachmaninov Piano Concerto no. 2 at the end of the first half of the concert, before intermission. As I took in the gold and light, statues and symmetry of the *Saal,* the symphony opened with Tchaikovsky's *Capriccio Italien,* a manic fantasy based on Italian folk songs, which the Moscow press of Tchaikovsky's day had labeled "cheap and coarse."

Besides those snippets of *The Nutcracker* that were difficult to avoid—particularly with a sister in ballet—the *Capriccio* was the first piece by Tchaikovsky I had ever heard. With the last three dollars of the money gifted to me by my grandmother for my tenth birthday, I had purchased a recording by Leonard Bernstein and the New York Philharmonic. With a strange mix of anticipation and fear, I had placed the record on the turntable. I'd been eager to explore this new world, yet fearful that it would disappoint as had so many things before. Would the price of admission be beyond my reach?

Nonetheless, the music's alternate resigned melancholy and ebullient hysteria had reached me in a way that nothing else could. Like meeting someone for what is supposedly the first time and then realizing that it simply cannot be the first time, the connection had been that comfortable. Coming home: being understood and accepted without having to become someone else. That was how Tchaikovsky's music had made me feel—and still did: that my anguish was not in vain; that there were others who felt this, too; that pain, when it is communicated, can change the world. Tchaikovsky's courage in the face of his pain, his ability to make it beautiful, had inspired me to become a composer. From the moment I had first heard the *Capriccio,* I had made it a personal quest to hear every piece Tchaikovsky had ever written and to read every published word about the man. This soon led to uncovering everything I could about the art of musical composition, until the parallel pursuits converged to chart my own artistic path. I had carried the pocket score of Tchaikovsky's Piano Concerto no. 1 in the deep recesses of my coat for three months before I began to write my own piano concerto.

I was certain that if I could have met Tchaikovsky, if he were still alive, we would have become best friends. I recalled reading in a biography of him how as a boy, he had once shot up in bed crying: "The music, the music, save me from it!" Upon being told that the guests had already gone home, and the music from downstairs had long since ceased, the little boy pounded upon his head hysterically: "It is here, *here!* And it won't leave me in peace."

I had felt a soothing shiver upon reading those words, for I had experienced the same sensation as a boy. Music would become a captive of my brain, railing against the edges of my sanity like a surge against a dam. It could not escape and, therefore, I could not escape.

I had also found it interesting that, like me, Tchaikovsky had not been a prodigy, not seriously considering music as a profession until he reached his twenties. Certainly, I had also read about his sickness: manic-depression. At that time, I could not have known how similar he and I truly were . . .

It was exciting to hear this piece performed live by the same conductor I had first heard on a recording many years ago. The interpretation I now heard was only slightly more subdued than that of the younger Bernstein. Although the man seemed tired and timorous, the music was energetic and vibrant—even wild.

The *Capriccio* came to a frenetic close, which was followed by equally frenzied applause, as fitting as a bitter stout chasing a shot of bourbon. It seemed as if the music had flowed naturally into the audience, so that their enthusiasm became another aspect of the same sound. A shiny black Bösendorfer was rolled center stage, and again, the orchestra tuned—this time to C minor. I watched the conductor. His poise and confidence belied all the agony it had taken to achieve his position. No doubt, few in the audience had the insider view, as did I, of what was required to earn the right to stand on that podium.

The number of orchestras prosperous enough to employ a full-time conductor across the entire world only tallied in the low hundreds. Competition was, therefore, ferocious. Simply to do his job, a conductor needed to be at least competent in English, German, French, and Italian. Although most conductors' primary instrument was piano, knowledge of all orchestral instruments—

their technique and nomenclature—was only the beginning. The microcosm of the individual voices and the macrocosm of the score had to become instinctive. Besides, it was never just about the music. Managerial skills of a top executive plus the patience of a kindergarten teacher—musicians were a temperamental lot—were a prerequisite. Most important was an attribute that could not be learned or taught—that rare brand of intangible charisma that softens the most brilliant, headstrong people into acknowledging the maestro's superiority—or at least, into admitting that he has much to teach them. This makes people step aside and let him pass while they enjoy the show, content to be whatever small part they can in his light. Without this, no amount of genius could do the trick. How does one achieve this? Through the totality of experience: the music cannot simply wash over you like bathwater. It must penetrate deeply, carving away at your insides until it creates something new.

The quintessence of all these qualities was Bernstein. His charisma had made him a citizen of the world, as equally at home in London, Prague, Sapporo, or Tel Aviv as in New York. He not only broke all the rules—he shattered them, becoming the first American-born music director of a major orchestra in his own country at a time when no one who mattered believed that a great classical musician could be born outside Europe. However, he didn't stop there: he became the first American to conduct the Berlin Philharmonic, the Vienna Philharmonic, the London Symphony, and the Royal Concertgebouw. In 1953, he was the first American to conduct opera at La Scala in Milan. He spoke five languages fluently and could exchange pleasantries in a smattering of others. At least six cities around the world gave him ceremonial keys, including Oslo and Vienna. He was an accomplished communicator, teaching at Brandeis University, writing four books about music—even giving a series of lectures at Harvard on poetry. He won eleven Emmys, one Tony, the Grammy Lifetime Achievement Award, and the Kennedy Center Honors. During his career, he made more than 400 recordings. What made the difference between someone like Bernstein and the average wannabe? Magnetic personality, for one thing, and mind-boggling enthusiasm for one's craft. It was also the ability to make people from all walks of life feel comfortable, even enhanced, in one's presence: presidents must feel honored; average citizens must feel inspired, not patronized. There was another element of success, something my father always said of my mother when I asked whatever had attracted him to her in the first place: seemingly infinite malleability—the ability to be at home everywhere, to act appropriately in any given situation.

It was also important to understand that life and art cannot be separated. Like any lasting relationship, each must nourish the other. Attempting to leap back and forth between the two, many artists have fallen into the abyss. One must learn to embrace the sprawl, living with a foot in the mud and a hand in the clouds at all times. The ordinary and the extraordinary must coexist within the soul of the artist, who must, in turn, coexist with contradiction: what is and what could be. The distance between what has already been created and what is yet to be created is too microscopic to measure. It is a single spark of light, of love, igniting being. A split second of connection is all it takes to make something exist that did not exist before. The problem is that the human mind magnifies this tiny interval into a perilous cavern.

However, when art merges with life, there is less room for fear. Greatness lies in the ability to connect one's art to the human experience. Being truly alive teaches one how to create art; being truly in one's art teaches one how to live. A true musician feels music with all the senses, which is why Beethoven could continue to compose after becoming deaf. Music that people care about, that moves the world, connects the abstractions of sound to one's own thoughts, feelings, and experiences of the world. This makes everyone feel less alone.

As Bernstein wrote: "Life without music is unthinkable, music without life is academic. That is why my contact with music is a total embrace." He was not afraid to reflect his life in his art, to integrate his senses and experiences for the world to see. For example, some argue that Bernstein's style changed after the death of his wife, that it became more somber and nostalgic. I think he just became more of what he had always been. In the end, art is about acknowledging what one is.

The scope of one's repertoire, the knowledge of oneself, the passion of one's commitment, and the ability to communicate this knowledge and this passion without making others feel less of themselves—these are the qualities that bridge the gap between brilliant artist and famous artist.

Now, one cannot deny that there is also the element of being at the right place at the right time. Bernstein came upon the scene at the same time as did television. He was able to leverage the new medium as a way to educate the American public about classical music.

When I was a kid, purchasing an LP with my last three bucks, I saw in Leonard Bernstein not only everything I wanted to be, but also everything I already was. Like me, he was a first-generation American Jew with a practical father who did not believe in music as a viable career option. Leonard's Aunt Clara gave the family her piano when she was forced to move after her divorce. As Leonard later wrote, he was instantly captivated by the instrument and "made love to it right away." Since his father would not pay for piano lessons, Leonard gave lessons to others in order to raise money for his own. Eventually, he attended Harvard—probably as a concession to his dad—but instead of taking up a typical Ivy League pursuit such as business or law, he majored in music.

Despite—or because of—his all-American persona, he never forgot his Jewish roots. He contributed greatly to the worldwide acceptance of the music of Jewish composers—for example, Aaron Copland—and created strong ties with the state of Israel. Two of his symphonies—the *Jeremiah* and the *Kaddish*—derived from his heritage.

His third symphony, the *Kaddish,* had been a personal favorite of mine ever since the night I had heard it on the radio. I had been burning the midnight oil composing my own music when I heard this provocative piece for the first time. Bernstein's signature orchestration, alternating between tonality and atonality, carried the eerily candid rail against death to an ennobling conclusion.

The symphony is drama set to music with Bernstein's wife, the Chilean actress Felicia Montealegre, narrating a one-woman struggle with God. She takes God to task for allowing man to deny the feminine, when it is the feminine that is closest to God, the feminine that is most directly created in his image. The pain of creation is woman's purview: only she can teach man to "suffer and recreate."

Felicia's personal anguish is evident in her interpretation. It is as if she were saying: "I am not invisible!" No doubt, Bernstein contributed much to her anguish, carrying on a five-year affair, which eventually culminated in his abandoning Felicia to live with his lover. Although he returned to her a year later, she was already sick. Several months after they had gotten back together, Felicia was diagnosed with lung cancer. One year later, she was dead.

Such an outcome illustrates how much responsibility a man has for a woman he loves—or pretends to love.

Such thoughts chipped at my self-image. I had always wanted to be better than the average man. What would I be if I left Gina for Dawn? Just another schmuck, that's what. Gina was not the most stable, self-possessed person in the world. How could I live with myself if my actions caused her to self-destruct? In many ways, I owed my survival to Gina. Before I met her, my confidence was at an all-time low. Although I liked to think that I would have persevered in my art without Gina's encouragement, contacts, and influence, I could not honestly say this would have been so. And without my art, I may very well have checked out. Truly, I loved Gina—just not in the way I loved Dawn. I never imagined Gina having my child; I didn't know why. That connection, that energy just wasn't there with her.

Also, I had never made myself completely vulnerable to Gina, never shared my deepest insecurities about my art, my ultimate darkness. I didn't let most of the world in—most people thought I was just this easygoing, straightforward guy, brimming with an almost naïve optimism and a love for all people. Little did they know that I believed in nothing, expected nothing. Only Dawn knew this. Only Dawn knew that I was aware of my own genius, and it was all I could do to hide my disdain for those who were too stupid to see it. The questions Dawn had asked me that night on the roof had angered me because I couldn't answer them. Why was Gina's potential pain more important than Dawn's present pain? I could not answer that. Her questions made me feel less of myself. They forced me to face issues that I would rather leave buried, realities that were too painful for me to address. I cared about both of these women. I was comfortable with Gina. No doubt, she was less work—I could never hide myself from Dawn the way I did from Gina—but my soul did not leap at the sight of her. I knew I could never lie to Dawn, like I did to Gina, and get away with it, but just the thought of Dawn wired my mind and hardened my dick. And I couldn't do a damned thing to stop it. . . .

Dawn entered stage right and curtsied to the audience, offering a weak smile. She looked older, more tired—and even paler than I recalled. And yet, something else had changed—something that was difficult to define. She was beautiful to me in a different way—poised, aloof, unattainable. It was as if I were falling in love with her all over again. Then, it hit me: she had found "it." She had developed true star quality—presence. It is not always what you say, but how you say it. It is not always about who you are, but how you seem. This was true of Tchaikovsky and Bernstein—and, now, it was true of Dawn.

Depicting an image of supreme delicacy and imposing power simultaneously, her fingers hovered above the keys like a mother sparrow over a threat to her young.

The opening chords of the Rachmaninov Second were angry and monstrous: the left hand was expected to reach from the low F to the A-flat an octave above—a stretch of nine-and-a-half keys—while striking notes in between. Meanwhile, the right hand was occupied with a series of five-note chords, all spanning an octave. Dawn played the chords as they were written, in one authoritative strike; it was incomprehensible how her tiny hands could accommodate such vastness.

I once saw a sculpture of Rachmaninov's hands in some museum, during one of the many tortuous family vacations I was subjected to as a child. His hands matched the vastness of the chords he created. In fact, all his piano music suggested that he believed everyone had the hands of a giant—or perhaps he only wrote for himself, to stretch across his own vastness.

Many of the greats cannot manage these opening chords without a slight hiccup. In other words, they rapidly play each chord in two parts, attempting to give the illusion of uniform sound. Some pianists even turn the chords into arpeggios, or "broken chords." The notes of a broken chord are played in rapid succession, strummed like a harp (hence the term arpeggio, which is the Italian word for "harp"). Each note is played and held, with the next note following quickly behind, building upon the first sound, then the second, until the harmony is gradually revealed. The effect is quite different from "blocked chords," whose components are played all at once. It is like the difference between knowledge that seeps in cumulatively and insights that flash instantaneously, charging the senses.

Although her hands were probably half as large as the master's, Dawn had found a way to capture Rachmaninov's vision precisely. It's all in the details. It takes a great man or woman to even understand this, to be humbled by the "small stuff" to the point of enlightenment. No expenditure of energy is too great for that extra effort: the wrapped present, the shined shoes, the clean handkerchief, the linen napkin, the parsley on the plate, the five-minute wait before exploding into anger, the "just one more" attempt at making contact, the sliver of willpower that helps you turn your back on weakness . . . the loyalty to the artist's vision. The refusal to accept what is "good enough." Our lives are a series of little moments, small kindnesses, and even smaller slights that define relationships and delineate dreams. After all, the difference between a great artist and an ordinary mortal is all in the details of handling limitations. Ordinary mortals are oppressed by them, while great artists are inspired to create ways around them.

To create a way around this limitation of size when playing the Rachmaninov Second is more important than it might appear, for what follows this sequence of nearly impossible blocked chords is a series of actual arpeggios. Without the contrast, the whole effect of instantaneous versus cumulative would be lost.

The watery arpeggios serve as a backdrop to the orchestra's hum of the primary theme, producing a hypnotic effect. The muted passion of the humming made me think of the accounts of those who had supposedly died and then returned to life. Many of their recounts involved a journey through a long, black tunnel accompanied by a strange hum. I imagined that this humming would contain all the passion and regret of their entire lives crammed into a few minutes or even a few seconds. This was what the opening of the concerto felt like to me: spiraling into an alternate existence, yearning to escape the baggage of my former life, yet being reminded—painfully—at every turn, how short I have fallen of my ideals.

This went on for nearly three minutes until the tension was almost too much to bear, and the piano took over the theme—despite the orchestra's protest—embellishing it with stately octaves and sweeping runs . . . humanizing it. The orchestra gently prodded at the piano, like the forgiving deity, with an occasional string passage or oboe cry.

The passion, no longer muted, swelled in intensity. The emotion seemed to be struggling against some intangible force that attempted to suppress it. Suddenly, the orchestra assumed the theme. Then, the piano and the orchestra continued their debate, which soon became a duel—as was common in the concerti of the Romantic period—until the passion surpassed them both, pouring forth without inhibition. The dispute between the piano and the orchestra had echoed the struggle between the passion and its prey. Now, the two must join forces to save themselves from the indomitable passion.

I knew all about indomitable passion: my life was constantly in threat of being ruled by it—sometimes by the dark, sometimes by the light, but it was never just me. My biggest fear was losing control forever, of opening the floodgates and being unable to dam them, of spiraling through the black tunnel and never coming out the other side. . . . I had not heard Dawn play music of so much emotional complexity before. Despite the magnificence of the Mozart concerto (that I had heard her play at Peabody), it seemed like the intricate sketching of a precocious child compared to this: the difference between the concept of pain and the experience of it. Despite his brilliance—or perhaps because of it—Mozart kept his distance. I recalled that when Mozart's wife was in childbirth, he sat at the foot of her bed and quietly wrote the second movement of the *Haydn* String Quartet in D Minor. After the child had been produced, he turned away and wrote the third movement. Talk about distance. I imagined that Rachmaninov, on the other hand, would have completely lost himself in the intensity of the experience, would feel the pain, the struggle, and the beauty. He would process the experience for weeks afterwards, and only then, could it appear in his music, with all the rawness of blood and fire. All of this would take from him, exhaust his life force, but the result would be yearning, physical artistry, as opposed to pristine cerebral prowess. Ironically, the physicality would make it far more spiritual: the essence of impermanent man questing for the essence of permanence—of God, I guess.

Dawn was definitely more akin to Rachmaninov than to Mozart. She fearlessly embraced the passion and made it her own. Her romanticism was not weepy or self-indulgent; it was quietly strong. Her melodic lines were not gracefully legato but percussive. Her rests were just as clear as her notes: there was as much energy in the small silences as in the sound. "What is the sound of one hand clapping?" asked the master. Answer: the sound of one hand clapping. Sometimes, things are no more than what they are. Sometimes, it is important to choose to be in the now.

The emotion in Dawn's playing was a conscious decision: she seemed to have complete command of it; furthermore, she had confidence in her command of it. She was like the refined woman you meet at a party: without so much of a hint of her passion, you know it exists. You can sense it from across the room. Such a woman is far more enticing than the kind that practically sits there with her legs spread, saying: "Here it is."

As I watched Dawn's body become infused with the music, impregnated by it, I felt a strong desire to have a child with her. I recalled that no other girl had ever made me feel this way. It was a deep-set, primal desire to share the ultimate with this extraordinary woman. It gave me an erection just thinking about it.

A sharing of another life: that is what made the current life worthwhile.

Despite his angst for perfection, despite his imagined inadequacy and his actual mastery, Rachmaninov was now dust in his grave, just as I, despite my striving, would be, too. I did not want to waste my life in angst. But how to stop . . . how to stop? The music made me realize what a fool I had been, and yet, at the same time, it reinforced the sorrow of it all. The awareness of this dichotomy made my head hurt even more.

I suddenly realized that, lost in my thoughts as I had been, I completely missed the second movement. Oh, well . . . I never had much patience for the slow movements anyway. Tranquility was such a bore.

The third movement began with a flourish. After the orchestra's introduction of a mere twenty measures, the piano hit the ground running with a *quasi glissando*. A *glissando* is when the pianist plays a rapid scale passage with one thumbnail, and *quasi* means "as if." So, together the two words mean to play a rapid scale passage as if you were playing it with only one thumb. In other words, with two hands, the pianist must achieve the glassy slur of an indefinite one-finger run.

The third movement is a march of fortitude—both in its message and its requirements—featuring rapid triplets, eighth notes in thirds, fiery chromatics, taut passage work, and more of those murderous chords for which Rachmaninov has become notorious among performers. The music is the triumphant song of a man who overcame his demons. In 1897, Rachmaninov plummeted into severe depression due to the failure of his First Symphony. This depression lasted three years, crippling the composer inside him. Finally, in 1900, he wrote the unaccompanied anthem *Panteley-tselitel* and most of the love duet for his opera, *Francesca da Rimini,* but when he began work on the Second Piano Concerto, he became frozen with self-doubt. In desperation, he made an appointment with Dr. Nikolay Dahl, famous for his results with hypnosis and suggestion. For three months, Dr. Dahl treated Rachmaninov with direct suggestion: "You will begin to write your concerto . . . you will work with great facility . . . the concerto will be of excellent quality." And so it was: the Piano Concerto no. 2 was an immediate success at its world premiere in Moscow in 1901. The demons had been conquered.

I had the sense that Dawn, too, was conquering her demons upon the stage. Her playing had a desperate quality that was somehow liberating to behold—like she was taking on the demons of the entire audience, allowing herself to become deranged so as to be exorcised by the equally demanding black monster before her. Was the trade-off worth it?

She looked as if the price had already been too high. There was a hollow intensity about her that was downright frightening, that made her seem unapproachable. She was beautiful, yes, but beautiful in the way that museum porcelain is beautiful: awe-inspiring—but cold and forbidden to the touch.

Although, based on size alone, I could crush her fingers in one of my bare hands, they seemed powerful enough to strangle me from across the room by sheer projected force.

The pallor of her skin contrasted with the soft blackness of her velvet gown and the shiny blackness of the Bösendorfer. Although she was delicate, she exuded only power. Despite her thinness, she had curves, which the gown certainly did not hide. I knew from experience that those curves were off-limits, but this knowledge did not prevent my wanting them.

The percussive clarity of her feminine power—the way she made Rachmaninov her own—made me want her even more. Yet, I knew her body would never be enough to satisfy me; I also wanted her soul. . . .

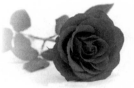

chapter 13: DAWN

November 1988
one hour later

"We have to stop meeting like this; I'll start to think you're a groupie," I said with as much poised indifference as I could muster. I was so glad to see him my insides ached.

"Do classical musicians have groupies?" Paul asked with a half smile.

"Hmm . . . I hear Joshua Bell does, and that blonde violinist—you know, the one who looks like she was poured into her bra . . ."

"You're not exactly wanting in that department," he said as his eyes dropped to my breasts.

"But I don't shove them in everyone's face."

"That's true."

"So," I redirected, unable to restrain my curiosity any longer. "What brings you to Vienna?"

He shot me an incredulous look. "I came to see you—um, to see you play, that is."

"But why? Besides, my booking was last minute. How did you hear about it all the way from Bern?"

"Ah . . . a magician never reveals his secrets."

"Is that all I'm going to get?"

"For now."

We crossed the Bösendorferstrasse, heading toward the Kärntner Ring.

"Where are we going?" I asked.

"Have you ever eaten at the Hotel Imperial?"

"Not recently," I replied curtly. I had no desire to reveal to what lengths I had to go to receive this booking.

The Imperial was one of the most expensive places in Vienna. Heads of state stayed there, along with anybody else who was rich and famous and preferred elegance over flash. I had dreamed of staying there—or at least, eating there—but never had.

I didn't ask if he could afford such a place. After all, Gina came from money. The idea of Paul buying me dinner with Gina's money was a little weird, I must admit. Nonetheless, it gave me a strange satisfaction, which, in turn, made me feel guilty. I decided not to ponder it.

As if reading my mind, Paul offered: "This is a special occasion, after all."

Erected between 1863 and 1870, the Hotel Imperial was originally the residence of the prince of Württemberg. It became a hotel in 1873. This palace-turned-hotel had the reputation of treating all its patrons like royalty, with its rooms of rich fabrics, nineteenth-century antiques, crystal chandeliers, and original art; its hallways of brass, marble, and mirrors; its balconies with views of the Musikverein and the Ringstrasse; its tuxedo-clad room-service attendants and butlered suites. Wagner had stayed here, as had, more recently, the Three Tenors. Here, the past was always present.

I would have been content to eat at the hotel's Café Imperial, where many writers and musicians were said to have written great works, inspired by divine coffee. Even my great-great uncle, Gustav Mahler, purportedly frequented the Café Imperial. However, Paul clearly had his mind set upon the Restaurant Imperial, which was the quintessence of formality and old-world grace. The moment we entered, the fastidious host nodded in deference and promptly seated us. All of the tables were sufficiently spaced to afford privacy. I sank into the deep cushions of the high-backed chair, allowing my drained senses to be replenished. This was certainly the ideal place for it. Talk about ambience! The soft, billowy glow of taper candles, reflecting off the varnished wood that encased the room on all sides—including the ceiling—created a sensation similar to sipping a fine brandy. Yellow roses, linen and lace, and fine glassware adorned the table, while the well-captured eyes of brass-rimmed portraits surveyed the scene.

Taking in all this elegance—being reminded that humanity was capable of such beauty and discernment—was like rubbing a salve upon my soul, soothing the burning irritation. No price was too high to pay for this . . . even though it was only temporary.

The menu offered too many choices for someone as indecisive as I: traditional Viennese dishes alongside more exotic creations of Hungarian, Czech, Turkish, and Serbian influence.

There were even offerings that blended two or more of these cuisines.

I gave Paul a helpless look, but he just smiled and turned to our waiter, ordering, in Schweizerdeutsch, the *prix fixe* dinner for both of us and a bottle of *Dürnsteiner*, a naturally sparkling white wine from the Danube Valley, which he ordered *herb* or "dry." It was not uncommon for Austrians to sweeten their tangy wines in an attempt to make them more palatable to foreign tastes. In my opinion, in that case, one might as well drink a soda. Apparently, Paul felt the same way.

"The Swiss have gotten to you," I said dryly, in reference to his Schweizer syntax.

"Well, you know what they say: when in Rome . . . though it does make me feel a bit unclean . . . when I think of what the Swiss did to our people during the Holocaust—neutral, my ass!"

I looked down in dismay, thinking of all the Jewish assets that had been seized by the Nazis and hidden by the Swiss, while the Swiss played innocent. My own family had been victims of such self-serving ruthlessness.

"Let's just have a nice dinner," I said softly.

"So, the best revenge is to live well—is that it?"

"Something like that." I tried to ignore the fact that he often seemed to reduce my sentiments to platitudes. Perhaps that was just a guy thing . . . whatever that meant. I tried to remember how happy I was to see him . . . I was also damned mad.

The waiter brought the bottle of wine and poured two glasses. I quickly drank the polite serving that he had poured and helped myself to another, more generous portion. I felt so much pain, I wanted to squelch it as soon as possible. What did Paul think he was doing, coming here? If he could not commit to me, what was the point? Yet, I could not deny that just being in his physical presence was soothing. I felt as though I had somehow never been complete before I had known his presence. But this was torture, for I could not have him. He was with Gina and would never be mine. If I had learned nothing, I had learned that. I wasn't a fool. Maybe I had been a fool, but . . .

I looked directly into his eyes and probed: "Does Gina know you are here?"

He evaded my gaze. "No—there was no need."

"No need?" I persisted. "But why not tell her?"

He began to look angry: "You know why."

"No, I don't. If you and I are just friends, after all, why can't she know? Why can't you come visit me in the same way you would visit one of your guy friends? Why should she be jealous if we are just friends?"

"Oh, c'mon! You know it's complicated."

"I'll bet."

"Yeah, yeah, I know . . . it's all my fault. I am just a sleazy man, and men always think with their dicks, right?"

"I didn't say that."

"No, but you meant it."

"It's amazing how your ego can't even handle a few innocent questions. I think I have a right to know what's going on. It's not all about you."

"Since when has it ever been about me?" he interrupted hotly.

"Why are we doing this?" I offered. "Look, I've missed you so much; I've thought about you all the time—I've ached for you, and now . . ."

"Oh, yeah, I'm the bad man. I'm ruining everything!"

"Will you stop? That's not what I said at all!" By now, the tears were streaming down my face. "No man has ever made me so pathetic. I have no pride where you are concerned."

"Oh, great! Is that supposed to be one of your 'compliments'? Is that supposed to make me feel good?"

"I'm just being honest. You know, when you criticize everything I say, it makes me more reluctant to open up."

"Well, maybe I really don't care. Maybe I'm sick of your nonsense."

"Then why are you here?"

Paul was saved from responding by the appearance of our waiter, who presented each of us with a large plate, covered by linen. I removed the napkin to reveal creatures of white, pink, and black resting upon glaciers of crushed ice. Lobster, salmon, and black caviar surrounded a single clam with open shell. Why, in such company, the clam should take center stage, I wasn't sure. I pierced the flesh of the main attraction with my tiny fork, dislodging the creature from its home. I nibbled around the edges and tasted ginger. I needed to be careful: ginger is an emmenagogue, and I was still bleeding.

We ate in silence, and I struggled to hold back the tears, not sure what to do next. Finally, I reached for his hand. "This is nice," I said softly.

He smiled weakly, squeezing my hand. "Yes, it is."

The waiter brought out the second course: apple soup, which I recognized as Hungarian from my travels in Budapest. The soup was very thick, and I sipped slowly from my spoon, savoring the taste of cloves, cinnamon, lemon, and dry white wine.

Next: a strange pudding, black in color, pungent in taste. I had no idea what it was called or of what it consisted. I didn't exactly like it, but it did provide quite a contrast to the creamy soup. I washed it down with the wine, which was hitting me hard.

"How long are you staying?" I asked without wanting to know the answer.

"I'm leaving early tomorrow morning," he replied without emotion.

"How long have you been in town?"

Paul looked up from his pudding with mischief in his eyes. "Since, oh, about an hour before your concert."

"What?" I nearly choked on my wine. "You came all this way just for one night?"

"I came to hear you play."

"But . . . you've heard me play before."

"Not with Leonard Bernstein."

"So . . . it's really Lenny you came to see . . ."

"Am I having dinner with him?"

"But traveling again tomorrow is insane. Why not stay at least one more day?"

"I—have to get back." He pretended to resume interest in his food as an excuse to avert his eyes from mine.

I knew better than to pursue this: he was saying he had to get back to Gina. I resumed interest in the wine. Tilted against the candlelight, the goblet looked like a crystal ball, bubbling with flecks of light. Did the secrets of my future lie in the pale yellow liquid? Without the effervescence, the landscape would be smooth and tranquil. How appropriate: there was always a bubble or two on the horizon to keep my adrenaline pumping. As I drank, the wine's tartness triggered a pulling sensation that traveled to my ears, biting like a lover—like I imagined Paul would do. I liked how the glass felt in my hand: hard and sensuous.

My reverie was interrupted by yet another course: *Tafelspitz mit Geröstete,* or "boiled beef with sautéed potatoes." Actually, what we had been served was a slight variation on the classic Viennese dish, for the accompanying *Schnittlauchsauce* (a sauce made from chives) was spicier than was customary. I tasted garlic and onions—an obvious Hungarian influence. The beef was tender and flavorful, and I ate with relish, thinking how much my body needed the protein and iron. I felt Paul's eyes upon me.

"I love to watch you eat," he said happily. "You really get into it. Most women don't. You give the impression of being delicate, but you're really intense; and you like intense things. It just amazes me how you can eat like that and stay so thin."

I shrugged. "I put a lot of demands on my body."

He nodded. "Speaking of that, where's your next gig?"

Now I was the one averting my eyes. "I—uh—don't exactly know, yet—exactly."

"Well, don't feel pregnant," Paul chuckled. "There's a lot of that going around."

"That's a strange choice of words. What do you mean?"

"You've never heard that saying? It means 'don't feel singled out.' A lot of musicians—even great ones—live hand to mouth."

"Except for *you,* that is," I replied, earning a look of surprise. "Well, you do seem to have turned into 'the chosen one.' Your name is all over the papers suddenly. You seem to have a lot of work lined up. How are you going to fulfill all those obligations while keeping up with your studies? Maybe I should hit you up for some jobs, Maestro!"

He drank from his glass, smiling mischievously. "If we worked together for any length of time, you really would become pregnant."

I laughed sardonically. "You *talk* bravely, but that's only because you live 900 kilometers away. It's all just a fantasy."

Paul shot me a sudden look of anger, which took me off guard. When he spoke, the intensity of his vitriol frightened me: "You're such a shrew! This is exactly why I hardly ever say or write romantic sentiments to you: I try to be cute, and you throw it right back in my face!"

"What?" I stammered. "I have no idea what you're talking about."

"Oh, yes! You are so sweet and innocent. It's all me; I'm the bad guy."

"I didn't say that, but when you're wrong, you're—"

"I'm always wrong according to you," he interrupted.

"Okay, when did I say *that?*"

"You don't have to *say* it!"

I tried to figure out what he was saying, but it was difficult. My mind was tired, and the effects of the wine had slowed down my world. I felt like a child caught in the middle of adult confusion. The effort to be understood was simply too much work.

Despite my silence, Paul continued to prod me, until I finally felt compelled to point out that if *he* were trying to remain quiet, while *I* attempted to keep the argument going, I would be labeled a bitch. Needless to say, this observation did not improve my cause.

I couldn't understand what had triggered so much anger— certainly not my flippant little observation. Although I knew that Paul's illness made him volatile and sometimes illogical, this knowledge did not assuage my fear. I felt like a little girl being chided by her father. I just wanted it to stop.

"Look, Paul, I'm really sorry for what I said," I ventured, even though I truly had no idea why I should be sorry. "I didn't mean anything by it; I certainly wasn't trying to 'throw anything back into your face.' Have you considered that, perhaps, your anger doesn't have anything to with me, that perhaps you're just angry at yourself for the way you feel about me? Perhaps you're just feeling guilty."

"Is that your idea of an apology?"

"I'm just saying——"

"Well, stop *saying!*"

"Look," I sniffled, trying to hold back the tears. "I'm really just trying to help, to get to the bottom of this so that we can bury it. I did say I was sorry . . ."

"Well, sorry is not good enough!"

"What am I supposed to do?" I demanded as the tears began to fall. I knew that my hormones were making me more emotional and obsessive, but here again, the knowledge did not help. "I can't take it back—I already said it! How can you be so mean?" I grabbed a knife from the table and poised it over my wrist. "What do you want from me—my blood?"

Paul quickly grabbed the knife from my hand as he nervously looked around the room. "Stop it! That is nothing to joke about! Lower your voice . . . people are staring."

"Now, you're worried?"

"Look, just stop it—okay? Can you do that?"

"Can *you?*"

"I asked you to stop and you keep right on going . . ."

"I stopped a long time ago."

"Whatever."

We were saved by yet another appearance in this seemingly endless procession of food. This time, it was some innocuous, flakey white fish that neither one of us could identify, covered in a multi-herb butter sauce. Alongside the fish was a nest of spinach leaves housing a dollop of caviar. Paul and I both looked at each other with wide eyes and simultaneously burst out laughing.

"How am I supposed to eat the babies with their mama watching?" I asked.

"Or vice versa," Paul deadpanned.

"Well, the babies *are* only eggs, but still . . ."

"Sounds like pro-life versus pro-choice to me: when does life begin—when the egg is fertilized or when it hatches?"

"Well, I never really cared for caviar, anyway—too salty." The truth was that salt, since it triggered water retention, made the emotional symptoms surrounding my period much worse. Unlike many women, my oversensitivity continued into the first few days of bleeding.

"Now, *there's* a digression if I've ever heard one, and not a very good one, I might add."

He was right, but I didn't care: we were laughing again. The truly funny thing was that I hadn't really been angry—only sad. I had given up anger a long time ago. I simply didn't have the energy to spare. I wished I could do the same with sorrow: just decide not to feel sad. But sorrow had such deep roots within my soul that I could not cut it out without removing part of myself.

Why was it that men were so often comfortable lashing out in anger, while women usually turned those feelings inward until they became depressed?

I also wondered why Paul seemed to feel he deserved a pat on the back for being a good man. He acted like he deserved a trophy for not jumping my bones or for being torn up about loving two women. Shouldn't that be a given? We women were continually tying ourselves up into knots, worrying about how our actions would affect other people. Why should a man be considered special for considering these things? I suddenly realized that it had been naïve of me to believe that just because Paul pursued me, he did not "truly" love Gina. It had been naïve of me to think that a man could not really love two women at the same time. . . .

At last, the end was in sight. The waiter presented us with the swirling, symmetrical, sugary epitome of decadence: the Imperial Torte. It was difficult to create a famous dessert in a city that viewed them as art, but the Imperial Torte was one of the best. It was just the right blend of creamy smoothness, substance, and sweetness, subtle in a way that only the Viennese could manage. With each bite, I could feel my eyes rolling back in my head.

The two strolling violinists, whom I had scarcely noticed previously, suddenly stopped at our table. They began to play *Dein ist mein ganzes Herz*—"Yours, is my entire heart." The melody was lush with longing, soaring with selfless abandon. We both became misty eyed as we mumbled the words:

Wo du nichst bist, kann ich nicht sein.
So, wie die Blume welk
wenn sie nicht küßt der Sonnenschein! . . .
Sag' mir noch einmal, mein einzig Lieb,
o sag' noch einmal mir: Ich hab' dich lieb!

(I cannot live without you.
I am like the flower that fades
without the kiss of sunshine! . . .
Say it once more, my one and only love,
say it once more: I love you!)

We knew it was time to go. Paul paid the obscene check, and we exchanged the timeless fantasy of the hotel for the finite reality of the dark night.

It was not yet cold, but there was a bite in the autumnal air—a dampness that prodded painfully, seemingly with the purpose of invading one's bones, of chipping away at that sense of *Gemütlichkeit,* for which the Viennese are so well-known. The alcohol coursing through our veins lessened the effects of the dampness, but it was still there. We proceeded along the Ring and turned right on Akademiestrasse, crossing the Mahlerstrasse and two other cross streets, until we came to the Wiener Staatsoper (Vienna State Opera). From across the street, the building looked like an old sleeping monster with hollow eyes, out of time and place against the modern traffic that populated the surrounding Ring, as if the town folk had simply decided to let the creature remain for fear of inciting its anger. Yet, the house was still vibrant with cultural life. I had seen several productions there with my father, for some of the artists that he represented had sung in leading roles. The present-day building was only a shell of what had once been: the bombs of War World II had made sure of this. The front façade had actually survived and whatever could be restored to the original style had been; however, the former opulence of the interior could not be recreated. As for the original, Emperor Franz Josef had not found the finished product imposing enough, and the architect—unable to handle the criticism from his superior—had committed suicide. Supposedly, the gentle emperor, afraid of triggering a repeat performance, had thereafter limited his commentary on artistic projects to the formulaic: "It was very nice; it pleased me very much."

It seemed incongruous to see "yield" signs and taxicabs against this paragon of the archaic. It was sad to see such cleaving to tradition, such defiance of progress. Yet, it was also reassuring. After all, I, too, was an example of such cleaving to the beauty and grace of a former time—and so was Paul. We both devoted our lives to the preservation of classical form. We both longed for permanence in a world of impermanence.

I could feel the energy in the old building, and I sensed that Paul felt it, too. I leaned against a blank space of wall between an imposing door with Roman arches and a placard that announced *Herbert von Karajan Platz* in red letters, aligning my back with the cold stone, pressing my palms against the wall. Breathing in deeply, I merged my pressure points with the building, and my mind flooded with images: past performances, powerful personalities . . . moments of intrigue, passion, violence, and betrayal. Were these images the drama of human life or merely the operas themselves? I suddenly realized that I could only feel the coldness on my back; I could not feel it on my palms.

Paul moved in close to me, gently brushing a few stray hairs from my face. "Gosh, you're beautiful," he said. "And I love your smell."

"Do I have a smell?" I asked.

"Of course. Everyone does."

This was logical, but I could not remember noticing anyone's smell the way I noticed his now. I loved his smell, too.

He pressed against me, and I could feel his hardness. A warm, tingling sensation began in the center of my being and worked its way downward until I could even feel it in my knees. My insides felt soft and pliable—open. Mixed with these pleasant sensations, however, were different shades of fear. I pushed him away slightly.

"Paul, please . . ."

He stood back for a moment and just looked at me. Then he held out his hand: "C'mon, let's walk."

The roof of the opera looked strangely alive against the dark sky, which was beginning to look ominous. My legs felt heavy and as I took his hand, I fell against him.

"Are you okay?" he asked, quickly grabbing my upper arm.

"Just a little . . . unsteady," I replied in an uncertain tone.

"I knew I shouldn't have let you drink so much."

"I'm a big girl. Anyway, it won't last forever," I replied, smiling slightly, as we continued toward the Burggarten. Somehow I knew that my strange sensations had nothing to do with the wine.

As we reached the lush parkland, flanked by Hofburg extravagance, the rain began. Soon it was pouring, and we scurried toward the nearest building, taking cover under an arch in front of the Museum of Art History.

"Have you visited the museum?" I asked.

Paul shook his head.

"Well," I offered, "it is probably the most diverse collection of art in all of Europe—far more than the Louvre."

"That's not surprising," Paul replied, "considering that the Hofburg Empire was a melting pot of not only Germans, Hungarians, and Slavs, but also Belgians and Latinos. We think we are so unique in the U.S., but—"

"We have a lot to learn," I completed his sentence, enjoying the intimacy of doing so.

We stared across the landscape as sheets of rain created a wall between us and the outside world. Flashes of light split the rain in half. Suddenly, a building from across the courtyard leapt forward. I sucked in my breath. What was happening to me? Energy ignited my being as Paul's fingers touched my chin to turn my face toward his. For a moment, he looked intently into my eyes. Then he lowered his lips to mine. His kiss was gentle at first, skin brushing against skin, but it quickly turned passionate. As I moved my mouth, responding to him, I noticed that half of my face was numb. We moved further into the darkness as his body pushed mine against an inner wall.

It seemed that we could not get close enough. My body hungered for his in a way I had never known before. I thought of the first line of Edna St.Vincent Millay's poem, "God's World": "O world, I cannot hold thee close enough!" At that moment, Paul became my world, and I could not hold him close enough. His lips moved to my neck, nibbling, biting. He unbuttoned my coat and reached behind to unfasten my bodice. His hand then traveled around to caress my breasts. As he massaged my hardened nipples, I felt a tingling excitement in the center of my being that was difficult to transcend. "Here such a passion is / As stretcheth me apart," as the poem continued. All my life I had struggled to transcend my body, to live in my mind. The call of intellectual pursuits had directed my course. Now, my body called to me, threatening to drown out my mind. Moaning slightly, I reached for him, encircling his hardness, unzipping his trousers to meet flesh with flesh. The only other time I had touched a penis was in Karl's office, but this was different: I was in control, happily surprised at the velvety softness. Judaism had attempted to strip away my pride in being female, but perhaps God did care about women after all: the only reason to make this skin so soft was so that it would feel good inside a woman. As my hand moved slowly up and down, he became harder and wetter, until he, too, began to moan. I could feel my own wetness as his lips reached my breast . . .

"It is good I am leaving in a few hours," Paul whispered, nuzzling his cheek against my nipple. "We are on the edge. You know that. All I can think of right now is how much I want to make love to you. And I do mean 'make love' . . . I mean, I really do love you." He turned to circle my nipple with his tongue, sending wiry sparks into my abdomen. The heat within seemed to spiral like ripples in water, expanding—evolving. I felt like I was losing myself, and yet, I was becoming so much more. I grabbed his face between my hands, biting my lip so hard I tasted blood.

"Oh, God, Paul—I love you so much—more than I can even understand." It was the first time I had said it in *this* way: from a place of transcendence, beyond self.

"Ah, my little *rondine* . . ." He removed my hands from either side of his face and brought them to his lips, slowly kissing the length of my fingers. "I'll be in Bern at least until next year. Then I don't know what will happen in my life . . . and you're still such a girl. I don't want to hurt you."

But I was already hurt. I pulled my hands from his and looked away. We stood in silence, except for the rain.

Finally, Paul spoke: "I need to take you home; we should find a taxi."

I shook my head as I took his arm, leaning against him. "I like the rain; let's just walk." Actually, I couldn't care less about the rain, but I needed it to cool me off—and to mask my tears.

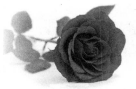

chapter 14: PAUL

May 1990

I couldn't believe I was going to see her again. I
hadn't seen her in well over a year, not since that crazy
night in Vienna—in the rain. We had written to one
another, but the tone had become cerebral, professional.

Since that night in Vienna, Dawn's career had
taken off. *Der Standard* had deemed her performance
"powerfully feminine and deliberate," and the *Wiener
Zeitung* had stated: "Wassmer's clarity of understanding brought the full emotional range of Rachmaninov's
expression to life." Such accolades had lead to
increased status at the agency, which, in turn, had lead
to better bookings. They had even extended her contract, and during the current season alone, she had
played all over Austria, Germany, France, Italy,
Scandinavia, and the British Isles. The tearing down of
the Berlin Wall at the end of last year had made the cultural richness of the former East Bloc more accessible,

and Dawn had even played a series of concerts in St. Petersburg "without an assigned escort" (as she had daringly stated in an interview with the BBC). I had no idea how much demand she was in until we tried to book her for our concert series and were given only two possible dates. Luckily, one of them fit our schedule. It was a twist of events I was happy to see: I had actually thought I was doing her a favor by requesting her, but her agency made us feel like they were doing *us* a favor by allowing her to play with us—"us" being the *Berner Symphonie-Orchester,* of which I was now assistant conductor under Dmitri Kitajenko. I had not planned to remain in Bern after receiving my master's last spring, but the offer had been too good to refuse. Since Maestro Kitajenko would not officially step into the role of principal conductor until the coming fall, he was still something of a freelancer. Therefore, his salary did not match his responsibilities, and he toured extensively as a guest conductor. This afforded great opportunity for me. In his absence, I was able to assume considerable authority, and I had conducted a far greater percentage of this season's forty concerts than most assistant conductors would otherwise receive. The timing couldn't have been better, for I had received a Guggenheim for the upcoming fall, allowing me to remain in Bern for the next two years to earn my doctorate from the *Universität.* The exposure I had received at the symphony had truly been the coup that had secured the grant, for it had showed my commitment both to music and to the cultural life of Bern. At the same time, Kitajenko's promotion would reduce my duties in the coming season, so I would be able to juggle both my assistant's position and my studies. Things were definitely looking good.

Thanks to a glowing recommendation from Hirsbrunner and my string of good reviews, I dare say that Kitajenko's respect for my musical judgment was so great that I could have brought Dawn in as a soloist even if her name had not become so well-known. Nonetheless, her recent successes made my task considerably easier.

She was going to play the Prokofiev Piano Concerto no. 3 here in Bern with me conducting. She had once said that she was saving this concerto for me, for us to play together.

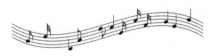

Dawn was late for rehearsal, and she arrived looking tired and distracted. Nonetheless, she was well put together in a long dark-blue cardigan over a well-pressed white oxford and long black skirt that accentuated her too-thin form. I actually wouldn't have minded seeing her gain five or ten pounds. Her hair was pinned up loosely, with wild strands flying every which way, which I found sexy. As she crossed the stage, I noticed that her left foot dragged slightly behind her. Amazingly, I noticed all of this out of the corner of my eye, for by the time she graced the stage, we were already rehearsing the short tone poem by contemporary Swiss composer Meinrad Schütter, which opened the program. The piece was difficult to understand, and the musicians were becoming restless. Being a composer myself, I felt it my duty to project a sense of dignity and respect concerning a colleague's work, but secretly, I longed to join the musicians in their jeers and snide comments. As is often the case in a symphony orchestra, many members did not take direction very well and required a firm hand in order to follow the through line of any piece of music. That being said, in this case I agreed with them: this piece made little sense, and we had no business performing it, Swiss national or no. In all fairness, Schütter had written some truly fine pieces . . . too bad this was not one of them.

Nonetheless, as soon as that was out of the way, Dawn would join us in the Prokofiev. Then, after intermission, we would conclude with Bruckner's Symphony no. 4.

At long last, it was time to rehearse the Prokofiev. Finally, a highly polished professional who could take direction!

In the Prokofiev Three, there is a rapid-fire dialogue between the orchestra and piano that requires a tight, precise rhythm. After a tranquil and brief introductory theme that begins in the woodwinds and quickly transfers to the strings, then accelerates as though it were being chased, the piano enters with a bite. It grabs the docile theme and turns it on its back, prodding at its underbelly to provoke its anger. A tug of war ensues: a violent emotional outburst that suddenly turns comic, like it is mocking itself. The piano's percussive chords, which sound almost like the indiscriminate banging of a defiant child, dissipate into the whimsical prattle of a clown. For all of this to make sense to the listener, the integration of the piano soloist with the orchestra needs to be seamless. It is imperative that the piano enter precisely on the correct beat.

I knew that Dawn knew this, but she did not do it. She came in late and remained behind, albeit only by a second or two—but that was too much. Then, her phrasing became muddier and muddier until I couldn't bear it anymore, and I called a halt literally in mid-bar.

"Let's try that again," I said. Turning to Dawn, I added: "You need to come in decisively, on the beat." She had neglected to bring a score—but soloists are required to play from memory, anyway. So, I removed mine from the stand in front of me and placed it before her. Then I carefully delineated the phrasing. She nodded in understanding, and I felt confident that the confusion had been cleared . . . until we tried again, and she made the same mistakes in the same places. When I stopped the music a second time, she looked confused, unsure of why we were repeating the same section: "But I did exactly what you said," she protested.

"No, actually you didn't. But we'll come back to it." After all, sometimes it takes a soloist a little time to become accustomed to the idiosyncrasies of the orchestra and vice versa, I told myself. However, later in the first movement, she sped up considerably, wildly, going way ahead of the orchestra in both tempo and emotion. Then in the second movement, there was too much delineation in the primary theme, yet in the variations, there was not enough. I noticed that her left hand was shaking uncontrollably. Her perceptions seemed skewed. All of a sudden, I was struck by an unsettling realization: these technical difficulties were merely symptoms of a much bigger problem. She was becoming too close to the piece, rooted in individual notes, unable to elevate her awareness. The realization was unsettling because, previously, her transcendence had been precisely what had set her apart. Finally, I called a ten-minute break and asked Dawn to meet with me in my small office.

"These four segments of the first movement are thematically unrelated," I said, using the score as a visual aide, "but they must *seem* interconnected, each naturally flowing into the other."

She nodded.

"They must become tighter as the movement progresses. This requires an increasing amount of restraint, not animation. Save the abandon for the third movement. It will have more impact."

"Yes, I see." Her eyes became wide. "I understand."

"Good. And now, for the phrasing." Slowly, we went over all the problems I had addressed previously. She acted like she was hearing them for the first time, asking many questions. After pulling out a tiny notebook from her side pocket, she fumbled around in her remaining pockets for a writing instrument—without success. I offered her my pencil.

"Thank you." She took the pencil and began scribbling furiously. "And what did you say about measure 23?" She had asked me about measure 23 at least three times before.

"Forget measure 23. It was just a dynamic marking. It is not that important."

She stopped and rubbed her temple, screwing up her face as though I had just asked her a difficult question. "I don't want to forget about it; I just want to get it right!"

"Great. That's all I want, too. In that case, there were some serious problems with your passage work in the second movement. . . . Are you listening to me?"

Dawn's eyes had begun to wander, and her demeanor had become anxious. "I'm just so worried I won't be able to remember those dynamic markings—and the phrasing," she said softly.

"But isn't that why you were writing it down?" I tried to reassure her.

"I still might not remember . . . that I wrote it down." She seemed frightened of her own words.

"Then why write it down?" I asked, more from a need to lighten the mood than from a need to know the answer.

"Because I don't know what else to do." Desperation became evident in her voice. "Sometimes, I feel like a deaf person. I know people are talking to me, but I can't understand what they say. I know it's important, but I can't find a way to remember. The concepts, the connections between things elude me.

Once, it all seemed so clear. Now, I know how Beethoven must have felt, gradually losing his hearing until he was no longer able to hear his music—or any music. But that was different. . . . I can *hear* with my ears, just not with my head. It's like what is going through my ears is not reaching my brain. Beethoven never lost his concept of music . . . the Ninth Symphony was a masterful, original conception . . . you said you were going to attend Bernstein's concert last December, when he played Beethoven's Ninth Symphony on both sides of the Berlin Wall, while people literally pulled it apart! Walls are intriguing symbols—blank, nondescript. The Berlin Wall reminded me strangely of the Western Wall, except people pray to the Western Wall. It is a symbol of hope. But people cursed the Berlin Wall. It was a symbol of despair, of separation. . . . Well, I was there . . . it was spectacular . . . musicians from East and West Germany and the four powers that had segregated Berlin getting together. Bernstein was magnificent! You know, his usual high-energy, schmaltzy self. Did you notice that he replaced the word *Freude* ["joy"] in the Schiller *Ode to Joy* text with *Freiheit* ["freedom"] . . . It was so great working with him in Vienna; I truly owe everything that's happened in the past year to him, to his confidence in me . . . remember that night in Vienna, after the concert, when we——"

"Look, we must get back. Are you clear on the passage work?" I interrupted, trying to redirect the flow of her mind. I certainly knew something about disconnected mental processes—I was bipolar, after all—but whatever was going on with Dawn was different. I just couldn't figure out how.

From her wounded look, I suspected that, in her female brain, she perceived my interruption as a way to avoid discussing our last meeting. However, the timing was purely coincidental; I just wanted to get back to work.

After scanning her notes, Dawn handed my pencil back to me with a professional smile. "Yes, I think we're good," she said with confidence. The sudden change in her demeanor was unsettling.

Admittedly, the first movement came out better—still not quite right—but definitely acceptable. The second movement, however, had its share of problems. Despite the overall slow tempo, the piano is given deceptively fast passage work, which demands the concentration of a diamond cutter. Since it is a theme and variations, it demands malleability from the soloist. Dawn had a difficult time switching gears: it took quite some time for her to transition from one style into another. The orchestra musicians struggled to follow her, but not without exchanging sidelong glances of contempt. Once again, I turned to my soloist: "Get with the program! Rehearsal time is at a premium here!" I heard the anger in my own voice and even though I knew that with Dawn's sensitive nature, it would only make matters worse, I couldn't pull in the reins. "You must wear many hats in this movement: athlete and artist, lover and warrior . . . once you get in the groove, you remain stuck! You're a trained professional. Why can't you trust yourself . . . and the music? Stop daydreaming and snap out of it!"

She froze, looking as frightened and confused as a lost child. Then her eyes filled with tears. "I'm sorry—I don't know what is wrong with me!" She covered her face in her hands and sobbed quietly. Some of the orchestra musicians smirked; some of them sighed; others made what were no doubt cruel comments to their neighbors behind cupped hands. Still others just stared.

I placed my hand on her shoulder. "Why don't you just take some time for yourself while we rehearse the Bruckner. Then we'll try again."

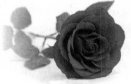

chapter 15: DAWN

May 1990
opening night

Non-musicians are always surprised to learn that every piano—even the most magnificent, well-crafted concert grand, easily worth six figures—has imperfections. Perhaps the high A sticks, or the lower register is a bit muddy, or there is a slight ticking in the hammer when F-sharp is struck *fortissimo*. Professional pianists learn to adjust to this. After all, we cannot just "bring our own" as does a flautist or violinist. A sense of humor helps. I recall that Guiomar Novaes, after being repeatedly betrayed by a single key that refused to sound in tune, stopped in the middle of a performance to thumb her nose at the keyboard. The audience loved it, and impending disaster became entertainment.

Such technical difficulties—even their potential—have kept me humble, proving that one can do everything right and still not achieve the desired result. Yet, since it is all about perception, if one can just have faith in the detour and stay open, the final outcome will offer more than he or she ever imagined. Or perhaps, it is more accurate to say that the outcome will *be* everything he or she imagined since nothing can become tangible without first becoming thought.

I am playing the same Steinway that Martha Argerich played here at the Münster, probably three decades ago. She, too, played the Prokofiev Third with Charles Dutoit conducting . . . Dutoit who became her husband. Agerich was considered one of the greatest pianists of the '50s and '60s. Now, many consider her to be one of the greatest of all time—right up there with Horowitz. Her recording of the "Rach Three" has become famous and deservedly so. In my opinion, her passion has been surpassed by no one. Had she left any of that passion behind? Had her sweat or tears permeated the ivory, leaving a hint of her magic the way some women leave traces of their perfume? Could I tap into this passion now, could I will it into rebirth through the power of thought? I certainly need help. There's an eerie clanging in the treble C. Since the concerto is in the key of C major, this is definitely a problem. I dread this awful reverberation before I even strike the key. Every time I know a C is approaching, I cringe, awaiting the electrical jolt that hits my spine with every clang. Yet, I must embrace this piano; accept its limitations, just as I would a child with dyslexia or a missing finger. Besides, I am far more broken than she. . . . *Oh! Another damned C!* It travels through my entire body, singeing all my nerve pathways until the sparks pierce through my fingers. Can the audience see the sparks? Will the sparks frighten them away? Can they hear the clanging or is it for

my ears alone? . . . *Oh, my God! There's an audience!* . . . I was drifting, but I shouldn't be drifting. I am onstage, performing one of
the most technically demanding concerti in the repertoire. I am
getting paid good money to be here, and people are paying good
money to hear me play. It was irresponsible of me to drift . . . I
have never drifted during a performance before. At least, I don't
remember having drifted, but I can't remember anything anymore—maybe I've always been like this and didn't know it,
maybe . . .

We're coming to the end of the first movement. I am suddenly taken in by the farcical quality of the final development.
Here comes the recapitulation. I'm supposed to remember to do
something here—what is it? How can I remember the finer
points of interpretation when I can't even remember the next
measure? I have been so afraid of getting caught in a loop because
the theme takes a different turn here than in the exposition, but
so far, so good. How can I play without thought? My body
remembers the music, even if my mind does not. In fact, my body
remembers it far better. *Accelerando!* Race to the end of the first
movement. Feeling Paul's eyes upon me, I turn my head only
slightly to take in his expression as he is conducting. Is that a look
of approval or disapproval? Am I doing okay? Would they regret
hiring me?

The second movement is too complicated: too much inter-
weaving, too much contradiction. The orchestra gets to keep a
fairly slow tempo, but many of my passages are fast.

That orchestral rehearsal was so embarrassing! I still don't
know why Paul became so angry; I did everything he told me.
He's the one who is stuck in the groove, if you ask me. I don't
understand why he had to yell at me in front of the entire orchestra. I certainly did not deserve that. What a temper! I hate when

people yell at me—especially men. It reverberates through my whole system, like the snap of a nine-foot Steinway D's string in an empty concert hall. At least, Paul and I were able to meet later for a one-on-one rehearsal in the practice studio, which has two pianos. He played an orchestral reduction for second piano while I, of course, played the solo. I wish we could have done that *before* the orchestral rehearsal, but unfortunately, schedules and space take precedence over art. During that session, he shared his monster with me, how he struggles to keep his bipolar disorder hidden, how he tries to use the insights his disease has given him without being consumed by it. As he said: "The second movement is comedy and drama intertwined, revealing a truth that all bipolar people know: there is not much difference between hedonistic glee and despair."

I know I gained so much from that rehearsal. Why can't I access it now? Every time I rehearse, it seems I figure out a new technique, a new method to overcome my difficulties—but when I begin work the next day, it becomes a new process all over again. I need to relearn what I was certain I would never forget.

Oh, no! I'm lost again! My hands are playing, but what are they playing? The stage lights are protecting me from seeing the audience but not from feeling them. They are not with me; I am losing them. What will I do? I need them to find my way, and yet, they are depending on me. Such fools! Don't they know I am going crazy? They are placing their trust in a madwoman! Besides, I don't even know them, as I sit in public privacy, thinking my own thoughts. Ah, but thoughts can become tangible! Perhaps they can see my thoughts, or at least sense them. "I think; therefore, I am." Does that mean I dreamed myself into existence? Does that mean I am creating this fear? How can I be afraid without knowing why? I'm an intelligent person—at least, I used to be—so it doesn't make sense. . . .

It took Prokofiev nearly ten years from first thought to bring this concerto into being. Ten years to write something that takes less than one-half hour to perform. But why not? Women spend days cooking meals that get eaten in fifteen minutes. . . . It takes me twenty-eight minutes to play this concerto now; I am not as fast as I used to be. Bryon Janis can play it in twenty-six minutes, nine seconds. Who cares? I am not trying to run the world's fastest mile—I am creating art, damn it!

I know that all of this is just my mind's way of distracting itself from its fear, but I have to embrace the fear, dive into the middle of it with my mouth open. That is what art is all about. I must be willing to drown in order to learn to swim, to shove my hands into the messy interior and pull it into the exterior. The irony is that one needs to transcend thought in order to make it tangible. I need to be present in the music the way I used to be. But it's not comfortable to be present now. There are sharp, stabbing pains in my fingers and in my back and neck. I keep practicing Czerny every day to work through it, but the pain does not go away. However, the pain is not the worst part: I'd rather feel pain than nothing at all. It's the numbness, like I'm feeling in my left hand right now—or rather, *not* feeling, I guess. How does one express what the sensation of lacking sensation feels like? I can't feel the keys! I can see that they are still there, but my hand does not know it—and yet, it is still moving. Oh, God, it kind of looks like a chicken with its head severed from its body: moving without feeling, purpose, or direction. I do not recognize this hand anymore, but I know it is mine; I must take responsibility for it. Yet, as hard as I try, I cannot make it mind. Now, I know how mothers of delinquent children feel. . . . Again, I feel Paul's eyes upon me. This time, I am sure he notices, for I feel his agitation. *Leave me alone!* I want to shout. *I have no room for your condemnation. I feel bad enough!* Mind over matter. Power of thought. Body memory. Come on! Surely one of these will work!

I am certain I have left out entire phrases of the second movement, but the orchestra is strong and Paul's direction is commanding. Perhaps no one noticed me. Oh, no, of course not! I'm only sitting in the center of the stage! Whatever made me think they'd give a damn about me with all this wonderful music going on around me, without me . . . in spite of me?

Wait! I must be fully aware of my body in order to transcend it. Transcendence will never come from a place of fear. I need to simply be . . . I have everything I need in the present moment!

I am playing the third movement. This is no longer about Prokofiev or Agerich or Paul Bailiff or the sea of faces behind the stage lights. It is about me: Dawn Wassmer. This moment is mine. No one else on this planet can bring this music into being in the way that I can right now. Only I have the power to bring the beauty of this abstraction into the concrete. Even Prokofiev has to release his creation into my hands, allowing his child to mature the way I see fit. I will play the way I want to play; the only way I can. Nothing else matters. . . . "This is the day which the Lord hath made . . ." I am fully alive for life's own sake; I am not here to meet the needs of those around me. I don't need their approval to exist—to evolve.

This movement is both playful and defiant, passionate in an aggressive, demanding way. It is a passion that is more cerebral than physical, more of illusion than of flesh. It could be the stuff of nightmare as well as of dream, except that it would be the kind of nightmare in which you never lose the realization you are dreaming. The terror is therefore safe, making bravery easy to feign. Then, the aggressive wave dissipates into an impotent stream as the enchantment of fantasy takes over. It is a somewhat erotic sequence, bordering on the grotesque—so different from the sincere pining, the Romantic abandon of Rachmaninov. This is the dreamy, self-deprecating, sometimes perverse, sensuality of the modern age. The melodies writhe like bodies, and their carnal enchantment reminds me of the lovemaking scene in Stravinsky's ballet, *Petrushka*. The romantic soul trapped within the body of a sawdust puppet named Petrushka is the perfect metaphor for modern man (and woman): metaphysical longing to feel something real trapped inside the plastic of privilege and material expectation. It is interesting how artists living in the same age seem to have their fingers on the same pulse, collectively revealing where man, where woman, is at that time. Their work often mirrors—even clarifies—one another's. For example, although Prokofiev did not complete this piano concerto until 1921, he had sketched the concluding passage of the first movement in 1911—the same year that *Petrushka* was first performed. . . . Here I go again: hiding in my intellect. *Get out of your head! It cannot save you! Only the music can do that.* . . .

My hands are alternating between pain and numbness. These arpeggios are brutal, and they must sound gentle. . . . Now, these chords must sound intense. The tempo is accelerating toward the finale. These hands need to really fly. *Get in the music— it will save you!* I am playing faster than thought, faster than feeling. I have found my lightness of being: I am sound! The pain does not matter—I was a fool to run from it, as foolish—and as human—as running from God's love. I have no idea where I am going. This is the most dangerous way to play, but is the source of all great performances. . . . Can I really make this energy work for me? Can I trust myself? I am opening the door of the wardrobe, entering the place "where the wild things are"—the center of creation.

Suddenly, I look down and see myself, my body rocking, my hands racing along the keys. I know that my heart is racing, too, even though I cannot feel it anymore. I am fully aware of the physical but unencumbered by it. I see the hammers of the Steinway pulsing furiously like the veins in the neck of a shouting man. I see the top of Paul's head, the sweat in his hair. And I see the audience. I have regained their trust, their temporal love. They are with me—their muscles taut, their eyes wide. I have this thousand-eyed monster by the tail, and I must bring him to climax by the sheer power of my illusion before he turns and devours me. How can I play when it is my body that is playing, and I have gone out of body? Yet, I know that I am playing better than I ever have in my entire life. I am an explorer, discovering uncharted land: aspects of this music and of my soul that I never knew existed. This is as new to me as it is to the audience. My life force pounds, leaps, guffaws as it races by, and I pounce, breathless, upon its fingers of light.

Paul is fully into the physicality of the performance; he has never looked sexier. I notice that my body is aching for him: I have returned to my flesh. I have become a synergy of myself: the sum being greater than the parts, than the soul or the body independently. I am electric with the magnificence of this life: how wonderful to have this music, this power, these senses; this physical desire for Paul, even this pain. How glorious to take this human woman form! I have been so stupid to sit alone in the darkness. The music will not relinquish: it acknowledges my existence and demands my commitment in return. It is persistent, wild. I feel like the girl in the fable, *The Red Shoes,* compelled by the shoes to dance herself to death. Could I have her courage?

Could I sever my feet to survive—or in this case, my hands? My mind is cooking; the sweat is flowing from my body. The beat of the tempo becomes louder and faster until its heart threatens to explode. But instead, it shatters fantastically into shards of light, into a splattering of C chords as redeeming as the sun. It is over. I stand quickly from the adrenaline and nearly fall like a fawn just learning to walk. Paul grabs my hand, and we bow to the audience. From the sparkle in his eyes, I know he is as high as I am. The audience showers us with applause, and the orchestra provides the thunder by stomping enthusiastically. Paul and I turn and nod to the orchestra, bringing them into the limelight, encouraging the audience to spread the love. Someone throws a bouquet of roses at my feet. Then another. I scoop them up, bringing them to my nose. Then, one by one, I liberate each flower, kissing its soft petals before throwing it into the audience, mouthing the words *danke schön*.

I play Prokofiev's *Toccata* as an encore. The mathematical precision keeps me in my head, while the driving rhythm reminds me of my body. This is good. I am no longer so enamored of my head that I cannot embrace my body. I am falling in love with my body, as if it were someone I am getting to know for the first time. Well, I guess it is . . .

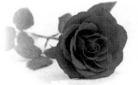

chapter 16: PAUL

May 1990
three days later

"I see the third movement evolving as a theater piece, an exquisitely twisted commedia dell'arte— whimsical but merciless. I'll bet manic episodes evolve in the same way—am I right? Bold and deluded, self-propelled and greedy, fascinating to behold but surreptitiously pernicious: Pagliacci's murderous jealousy seething behind his comical mask." Dawn seemed pretty convinced of her own insights as she turned to look at the fountain, whose sculpture of Moses pointed to the Second Commandment: "Thou shalt have no other gods before me." *Even God is jealous,* I thought. I suspected that Dawn was trying to find out more about my condition and that she was using a strategically placed analysis of our three-night concert series as a pretense. However, I didn't care. I was flattered that

she wanted to learn more about me—even if her interest was settling on a subject I'd rather not look at too closely. This was definitely better than our previous discussion: all the men that had
hit on her during her European tour. *I* was too jealous to listen to
any more of that. Besides, I loved her vocabulary. How many people used phrases like "surreptitiously pernicious" in ordinary
conversation? She clearly fit the stereotype of a classical musician:
erudite, refined, preoccupied with high ideals and the so-called
finer things. She was a dying breed, a throwback to an earlier
time. I respected that; I was often accused of being that way
myself.

"That's an interesting observation," I started carefully. "I
agree that Prokofiev is intrinsically theatrical. However, comparing a manic episode to Pagliacci's desperate acts is dangerous. It's
like saying that everyone with a mental illness needs to be put
away before they do damage to themselves or to others."

"That's not what I am saying at all!" She pushed her bangs
out of her eyes. "How familiar are you with directorial technique?"

I nodded. "Fairly so. I've always thought there were too
many parallels between directing a play and conducting an
orchestra to ignore this knowledge."

"Okay, great. Well, just as Stanislavsky created a play from
the inside out, tapping the interior of the actors, so, too, does a
manic-depressive create—or recreate—the world from his inner
tumult. Now, the real key: if only you could learn, like a
Stanislavskian actor, to manifest whatever emotion you needed at
will—more for the purpose of creating your own reality than for
influencing those around you—then you would be the master of
your fate . . . a kind of artistic Superman."

After I looked at her incredulously, she added: "It is not that different from interpreting Prokofiev."

"For one thing, the techniques of Stanislavsky could certainly apply to the interpretation of Rachmaninov or Tchaikovsky, since both of these composers require the performer to tap into his own emotional memory in order to bring psychological immediacy to the pathos of the composer's vision. However, this would not work for Prokofiev, whose conception of art seemed to be that of an outsider looking in. According to his wife, Prokofiev did not create from "inspiration," but from structure and discipline, keeping a huge file of fragments and themes to get him started each morning. He was a slow worker, but capable of juggling many projects at once because he maintained distance." I said all of this quickly, trying to mask the growing impatience in my voice. Why did she have to go off on these tangents and then not let go? "To stay with your theatrical metaphor, Prokofiev was more like the director Vsevolod Meyerhold, who believed that the overall unity of the performance composition must penetrate the interior. Meyerhold didn't have the patience for bloody excavations of the psyche. He preferred to create a structure wherein all the components contributed equally and just see where that led. And Prokofiev was the same way. His third piano concerto is a prime example—at least, in the way I view it and prefer to interpret it."

"Ah, but that just mirrors your own mode of survival," she jumped in excitedly, her voice getting louder. "You live in the structure; it's what keeps you going. In the surface construct of things is where you choose to remain, leaving the dirty treasures of the damp cellar for the more daring."

"What kind of nonsense is that?" I snapped, unable to control my irritation any longer. "Is this your way of saying 'I told you so,' that our conflicts at rehearsal were unfounded, as evidenced by your subsequent success at performance? Are you saying that I am too parochial to understand your 'daring' interpretation?"

"No, not at all," she said softly. "Where did you get a crazy idea like that?"

"Oh, so now, I'm crazy! I got the idea from you, from your own words! You don't even know what you are saying half the time, do you? Do you even understand how it affects people?"

"Yes, of course, but——"

"Oh, I know! You're so misunderstood. . . . Well, then, the problem rests with you: *you* need to choose your words more carefully if they're not revealing what you mean! I can tell you, from the receiving end, your words sound pretty damned clear!"

"Okay, okay, you win!" She walked over to me. Then, giggling girlishly, she toyed with my ear.

"Cut it out!"

"I love your ears . . . they're *so* cute!"

"My ears are not cute. Come on!" But it was difficult to stay mad at her: *she* was the one that was cute. Besides, it probably wasn't her words that annoyed me as much as the realization that her "from the gut" interpretation of the Prokofiev had thrown me off-center. My view of Prokofiev—in fact, of most twentieth-century composers—was that of an intellectual "structurist." This was a term I had coined to describe the very "living in the structure" of which Dawn had just accused me. Nonetheless, even if that were true, I would be in good company: Stockhausen, Schöenberg and the atonalists—even John Cage to a certain degree—had lived in structure, creating their music from a mathematical construct, rather than an emotional insight. But it was not intellectual hubris or "mental masturbation," as some called it, for the structure had merely been a tool—like any other.

They had used the exterior to access the interior. What annoyed me most about Dawn's theory was that she didn't seem to realize that her reliance on her gut was just another tool to reach the same result.

"Look, it *is* true that the audience loved your interpretation, and each night, the crowds seemed increasingly enthusiastic. But what they were really responding to was the physicality, the eroticism of your playing—not what you perceive to be your daring psychological excavation!"

She crossed her hands in front of her, grabbing either forearm as if to give herself support. She cocked her head to one side and studied me for about a half-minute. Then a gentle, knowing smile came over her face. "What happened to me on that stage, on opening night, was not psychological—or physical. It was metaphysical."

"Oh, so you're saying you had a *spiritual* awakening?"

"Hmm. It was more of an awakening to my body—so I can see why you might have perceived it as 'erotic.' I guess it was erotic in a way, but not in the way we normally perceive eroticism. It was more 'singing the body electric,' to quote Walt Whitman. It was a sudden awareness of *all* my bodies—energy, etheric, spiritual, *and* physical—an awareness that the physical is as important as all the others. It was an instantaneous knowing that I am far more than my mind."

"And this is news?"

"Well—in a way. All my life, I've suppressed my body. I've beat it into submission through rigorous practice and study, denying its hunger, tiredness, loneliness, and need to just play. I've denied its needs, thwarted its desires, and muffled its cries. Now it is angry. Now it is punishing me."

I was startled by her bizarre words: "What?"

"My body is doing strange things, feeling strange things." While she spoke, she paced, and I noticed that her dragging left foot had become a limp. Her entire presence projected nervousness.

"What is your body doing?" I asked.

"I don't know—strange things. Suddenly my hands go numb, or my foot gets a sharp pins-and-needles feeling, or my face hurts, or I can't focus my eyes. Sometimes, I'm trying to communicate something, but I can't formulate the words. Sometimes, I drop the pen I'm holding because my hand seems to have a mind of its own. My senses of taste and hearing are off. There is this creepy, itching sensation all over my body, but when I scratch, I realize that the itch is *inside* my skin, underneath somehow, and I can't get to it. And then there is this brutal, mind-numbing headache!" Simultaneously, she rubbed her eyebrow with her forefinger and her temple with her thumb.

"Sounds weird, but you know, everything you're describing could be nerves . . . nervous exhaustion, that is. It happens a lot with performers. I'm sure you've been under a lot of pressure. It's probably stress. Maybe if you get some rest . . ."

"Maybe." She shrugged, suggesting that she was not convinced. "Well, I *am* going to get some rest pretty soon—for nearly a month. I'm going home."

"Really?" I was genuinely surprised at my sudden feelings of almost panic.

"Yeah, I'm leaving for Lucerne the day after tomorrow to do a world première of an Edison Denisov piece. Then I'm off to Zurich to play a series of concerts at the Tonhalle with Charles Dutoit. I'll end the season in Paris, playing the Saint-Saëns Second with Daniel Barenboim conducting. After that, I'm headed for Baltimore. I haven't been there in over two years, and

I need to see my family. Besides, there is this little problem I need to rectify."

"Which is?"

"I don't have a degree." She made the *shush* sign across her lips. "Many people don't even realize it—not that I try to hide it. I just don't go out of my way to point it out. But Peabody has agreed to allow me to use portfolio assessment for my professional experience and CLEP, as well as other advanced placement exams for many of my academic subjects, which means I could have my bachelor's by next May!"

"That's wonderful," I replied with sincere happiness. Education was extremely important to me, and I was glad Dawn was prepared to finish what she had started. At the same time, I worried that she was spreading herself too thin.

"Won't that be tough with your concert schedule—or are you giving that up?" I asked.

"Give it up? Are you crazy? Of course, I will need to modify it, but Peabody is pretty understanding about a student's concert schedule, you know that. Most of the undergrads have active performing careers—maybe not quite as active as mine, but . . . Peabody is a professional training ground; they'll work with any student who is validating how great Peabody is with her own professional success!"

"Well, of course."

"And *then,*" her eyes danced, "in July, I'll be playing in the William Kapell International Piano Competition at the University of Maryland, College Park. I made the Preliminary Round!"

"That's wonderful," I repeated. It was, indeed, quite an honor. The Kapell, named after a brilliant pianist who had died tragically young in a plane crash, was highly prestigious, and first prize in such a competition was like a calling card to the truly elite. Dawn's announcement of her status was a much bigger deal than it sounded, for the "Preliminary Round" consisted of an impressive group, selected from thousands of pianists around the world, each with his or her own array of impressive credentials. The applicants were required to submit tapes of their performances of difficult pieces, representing each of the music periods—Baroque, Classical, Romantic, and Contemporary—to the jury. From that impersonal screening, only forty were invited to Tawes Theatre to play the exact same repertoire they had recorded. During this performance, the jury could stop the pianist at any time. The "preliminary" group was then whittled down to twelve contestants for the semifinals. This consisted of twenty-five minutes of music as chosen by the performer, a newly composed work as selected by the jury, and thirty minutes of selections from the two piano concerti that the performer had designated in advance for the final round—should he or she get that far. Only three pianists actually did "get that far." The final round—playing one of the two previously designated concerti (the jury chose which one) with the National Symphony Orchestra at the Kennedy Center for the Performing Arts in Washington, D.C.—was the only chance the participant had to play with an orchestra, since the selections in the semifinals were accompanied by a second piano. I had worked with several pianists who had competed in the Kapell. None of them had even reached the semifinals. By the way, as was true of nearly all music competitions, the jury did not have to award First Prize at all if they did not feel any of the contestants were "deserving" of such an honor. A pianist could, therefore, be considered the best player in the competition and still only win Second Prize. The whole thing was a brutal marathon, an Olympics of the piano. Admittedly, in light of Dawn's obvious symptoms of nervous exhaustion, I was more than a little worried about her subjecting herself to such an ordeal. A lot of good her month off would do!

"But what about the summer festivals here in Europe, wouldn't that be a better use of your time?"

"Not really. I've played that circuit for the past two years, and I'm still relegated mostly to 'B' orchestras—no offense. Anyway, my father has been trying to wrangle a contract for me out of Columbia Artists for over a year, but since I haven't placed in any world-class competitions, they've been, shall we say, less than enthusiastic. However, when they heard that I was competing in the Kapell, they agreed to sign me on as one of their artists! So, I have to do this! I already have concerts lined up with some of the best American orchestras next season—thanks to Columbia. As you know, the Americans will barely spit in your direction without a top agent."

I didn't respond, for I was too busy thinking about the irony of all this: the woman before me was a brilliant musician, who had played with Leonard Bernstein, for Pete's sake! She had been touring the European continent to rave reviews, and yet she needed to compete in some ridiculous spectacle to catch the eye of a top manager. Didn't they realize that these competitions were almost never won by the greatest artist, but rather, by the most competent technician, simply playing exactly like everyone else only better? How was it even good business sense to focus on these performers? I did not believe that concertgoers bought season tickets to hear technicians. In any event, I did not want to believe it. Nor did I want to spend any more of our afternoon together discussing it. So instead, I turned to Dawn with the words: "Come here, I want to show you something that I'll bet you didn't notice."

We crossed the cobbled square, known as the Münsterplatz, and reached the central portal of the cathedral. She sucked in her breath as we stood before the *Final Judgment.* The contrast between the peaceful, smiling faces of the saved, which filled the left half of the portal, and the screaming, twisted faces of the damned on the right was terrifying. Justice sat in the middle, surrounded by the Wise and Foolish Virgins and a group of angels. Above it all, presided the Archangel Michael with a sword in one hand and a scale in the other.

"Now if that doesn't make a person pray, I don't know what will," I said.

"Hmm," she grimaced. "People always create justification for their beliefs—or disbeliefs. If one does not believe in God—or at least, in a judgmental God—it's easy to dismiss this image as the theocracy's way of keeping the common man under its thumb. In that case, the person would do nothing differently. On the other hand, if one already believes in such a God, this sculpture would incite fear and guilt, thus compelling said person to drop to his knees."

"And which one are you?"

"Ah, but is that really the question? I mean, does that really matter? What's more important, as an artist, is whether or not I believe that art has the power to change anybody."

"And do you?"

"Only if they want to change."

"Ah, yes—the old free will . . ." I sighed.

"Exactly! But why not simply choose to pray—to be with God—for its own sake? Why not choose to 'do the right thing' just because it *is* the right thing? Why does it have to be motivated by a fear of punishment? If you do something 'good' simply to avoid being considered 'bad,' are you even doing any good at all?"

We were interrupted by the bustle of a mother and her two children. They, too, stopped in front of the sculpture, obviously taken aback. The mother was dark of hair and eye and probably in her mid-thirties. The children, who were also dark, were well-groomed. I couldn't pinpoint their ages, except that they were both younger than ten.

Finally, the little boy spoke: *"Maman, regardez les monstres!"* ("Mama, look at the monsters!")

His mother replied: *"Ils ne sont pas des monstres; ils sont seule-ment des hommes qui sont punis. C'est ce qui se produit quand tu n'écoutes pas ta mère!"* ("They are not monsters; they are only men who are being punished. It's what happens when you don't listen to your mother!")

Dawn and I exchanged a knowing smile.

Suddenly, the little girl spoke: *"Regardez, Maman! N'est pas que la dame qui a joué le piano hier après-midi? La jolie dame avec les doigts rapides?"* ("Look, Mama! Isn't that the lady who played the piano yesterday afternoon? The pretty lady with the fast fingers?") The little girl pointed to Dawn.

The mother smiled in embarrassment, gently cupping her hand over her daughter's tiny, erect finger. *"Ce n'est pas poli"* ("That is not polite"), she whispered to the little girl. Then she turned to Dawn and immediately switched to English: "I am sorry, Madame, but *did* you play piano in yesterday's con-*sair* here at le Münster?"

"Indeed, I did! Dawn Wassmer, pleased to meet you!" Dawn grinned like one of the children as she held out her hand to the little girl, who looked nervously at her mother.

"Go on," the mother prodded. And the little girl timidly wrapped her entire hand around Dawn's fingers, without actually shaking. Her face, however, was beaming. Then, the little boy grabbed Dawn's hand and shook it hard. *"Enchantée,"* he said loudly.

"And this is the conductor, Paul Bailiff," Dawn offered, putting her hand on my shoulder.

"Maestro," the mother nodded. The children seemed less than interested.

"My children eh-study piano," the mother offered, with the look of trying to reassure me that their fascination with Dawn and not with me was nothing personal. "Marguerite wants to be—great music-ee-enne!"

Dawn, obviously aware that the woman was having trouble, offered: *"Je parle français."* And they were off.

I moved away from the portal, letting the two women talk, taking the opportunity to enjoy the spring air. That was one thing about Bern: the air was deliciously clear, which was unusual for a European city, most of which were overpopulated. Despite its status as the nation's capital, with barely 130,000 residents Bern was more like a town than a city. Cars were forbidden in the Old Town, which sharply reduced pollution, and the rapid-flowing Aare River, with its tree-lined banks, kept the temperature down. And then there were the Alps. . . . There was certainly nothing like mountain air. I had become quite accustomed to it, growing up in Washington State. I recalled riding up into the Cascades as a kid, getting carsick in the back seat but still excited at the first sight of snow. I thought about the Seattle of my childhood: blue-collar edgy, dirty—comfortable. Filled with longshoremen, fishermen, and merchant sailors. I had heard that things had really changed. . . .

I had originally planned to ask Dawn to climb the tower of the Münster with me—but that had been before I knew how exhausted she was. It was the tallest tower in Switzerland and had a steep spiral of 254 stone stairs. If you timed it right, you could actually be up there when the bell tolled. It weighed over ten tons and positively rattled you to the bone—a humbling but powerful experience. This unsettling pleasure aside, the 360-degree view of the city of Bern and its pastoral surroundings, including the Alps, was enough to even make a guy want to go out and rent *The Sound of Music*. I knew Dawn would certainly enjoy it, but now I hesitated to ask her—especially since her feisty nature would probably compel her to climb the stairs just to prove she could. When I had asked her about her limp, she had hotly denied it and had made an obviously painful effort to walk straighter—but to no avail.

I glanced over to see Dawn standing in front of *Justice* with the two children on either side, while the mother took their picture. *Now that's an interesting shot,* I thought. *Does that mother realize she's depicting one of her children as saved and the other as damned?* I smiled at the absurdity of it. It was even more amusing to think of Dawn in the role of Justice, deciding their fate, like a master teacher who holds the future of her students in her hands. In any event, the little party looked like it was breaking up.

The two women shook hands, and the mother continued talking rapidly. I couldn't hear what was being said, but at last, she and her children disappeared into the cathedral. Dawn looked lost for a moment, turning to look this way and that. Finally, she spotted me and headed in my direction, smiling.

"I'm sorry about that, but those children were *so* cute! And their mother was very interesting. We actually had quite a conversation." She grabbed my arm, and we began walking around the square.

"So I gathered. What could you have possibly found to talk about?"

"Oh, life, music . . . she remarked on the Baroque façades in the square, saying that at that time, religion was so integral to everyone's life that all the buildings and art paid homage to it. Then I brought up Bach as a prime example: the purity of his expression, the clarity of his mind. Same was true of classicists like Haydn. Then came Romanticism—Chopin, Tchaikovsky, Brahms, Rachmaninov, and good old Beethoven straddling the fence with one foot in the old and one in the new. Then, well— it all got screwed up: man became too fascinated with his own misery, and then, where was God? The Romantics rebelled against the Baroque and the Classical forms, that is, God—as represented by religion. They were humanists who glorified man and his ego—his lust and his darkness. It's like in Thomas Mann's *Doctor Faustus,* when Kretschmar lectures about Beethoven and his inability to master the fugue. Well, Beethoven symbolizes the Romantic, self-destructive ego, and the fugue symbolizes the structure of religion. Beethoven can't grasp the fugue because he is too busy resisting it."

"Wow, you got all of that from that French woman and her two kids?"

"Well, in a way—she directed my thinking along these lines."

"That's all very interesting except for one thing: where do we fit in? How does contemporary art and music relate to God?"

"I guess I'd like to think we've discovered that God is not really separate from us after all, that we don't need to communicate through religion, that we don't need all these Biblical commentaries. Faith cannot spring from these externals—but we can't throw the baby out with the bath water."

"In other words, finding no use in religion is no reason to reject God."

"Exactly."

I loved the way she said the word, hanging on the first sylla-ble until it sounded like "egg." I was amazed how Dawn and I could discuss such things so easily, how our thoughts seemed to click, creating an intimacy of the mind that was much more entic-ing, more erotic than sex. Even talking about God with her could get me aroused. I wondered if she noticed the bulge in my pants.

"I've come to realize that all religions boil down to two basic concepts. I didn't even know I believed this until one of my piano students—a middle-aged Jewish woman who had fallen away from organized religion due to its subordination of women, as had I—asked me how I could radiate such peace. Well, without having to think about it, the answer simply flowed from my mouth. I told her that I kept it simple, that to know God and find peace, there were only two things she needed to do."

"And what are those two things?" I asked, wondering when she planned to get to the point.

"First, to truly love other human beings. Second, to have the courage to live your destiny. Judaism, Christianity, Hinduism, Buddhism—you name it—they all come down to those two things. If you truly love God, you will respect and care what hap-pens to other people because you realize that they are just another aspect of yourself. Also, you will not throw your life away because that would be like slapping the God you love in the face."

We walked in silence after that, enjoying the presence of being: the cathedral, the square, children, each other . . . life.

"Of course," she abruptly continued out of the blue. "That might be too idealistic—the idea that contemporary artists have a, shall we say, more *evolved* handle on God. I mean, take Prokofiev's Third, for instance . . ."

And then, something eerie happened. Dawn repeated the exact same line of logic she had used to open our earlier discussion about the Prokofiev. She acted as though she were making these statements for the first time, with no apparent recollection of our earlier conversation. I felt a slight chill go up my spine. How could she be so forgetful and yet so brilliant? Not wanting to repeat the same argument from before, I gave her little feedback, curious to see where she might end up with little encouragement. I could never have predicted it.

"Overall, the concerto is pretty sexual, but not in a loving, healthy way. It reminds me more of a lonely genius masturbating in his disheveled room."

"What?" I burst out laughing at how her statement could be so bizarrely on and off the subject at the same time.

"I'm serious. Don't you see that?"

"Well, don't knock masturbation. It's come in pretty handy—since Gina left."

Dawn stopped walking. "She—left?" There was anticipation in her voice.

"Yes."

"But—when? Why?"

"About six months ago. Does it matter why? She's gone, and she's not coming back." I didn't want to go into all the arguments or Gina's impatience with my mood swings and aloofness. Or the time Gina found Dawn's letters. Or the mutual colleague who told Gina he had seen Dawn and me leaving the Hotel Imperial, arm-in-arm. It was too draining.

For once, Dawn took the hint. "Oh," was all she said. Then she giggled. "*Come* in pretty *hand*-y! Hah-hah!"

I shook my head. "You really are weird."

"And you love it!"

"I never said I didn't. . . . Hey, let's go check out the Münsterplattform." This was my solution to the tower issue. The platform was a buttressed terrace on the south side of the cathedral. It did not reach the looming heights of the tower, but it did provide an excellent view of the river and the hills. Not that it mattered where we were. After all, I had supposedly been showing her the sights, but all we had done was talk. We could be anywhere together, and it would be special. The "being together" was the special part. The rest did not matter. For me, the locale was not the main attraction—she was. Yet, I did want the next few moments to be particularly special.

"This really is beautiful," she sighed, looking out over the Aare, breathing in deeply.

"Would you believe that the Protestants once used this terrace as a dumping ground for all the Catholic icons they felt it their duty to dismantle?"

She just smiled and leaned against a chestnut tree. "Why is there a net under the parapet?" she asked.

"Oh, several people used this spot as the launch pad for their final dive. I guess someone decided that the net might deter those of a similar mind. What do you think? Would this be a good place to die?"

She shrugged. "I don't think any place would be a good place to die." Then she turned to me with intense eyes, taking one of my hands in both of hers. "Why did you do it? Why did you try to kill yourself?"

I searched her face for curiosity but found none. There was only concern, and it was painful. So painful, in fact, that I pulled away. "Oh, I don't know; I was having a bad time. I was coming down from a manic high. There is nothing more depressing after a manic high than ordinary life. I've never wanted to be ordinary.

I had all these visions of what I wanted to be in my life, where I wanted to go, but I couldn't see a way of getting there. I felt so worthless and trapped in my worthlessness. It seemed that nothing could ever be as bad as that feeling, that I would do anything to make it stop."

"But no one noticed that you were in trouble?"

"Evidently not."

"But what changed? What made you give life another chance? What made you stick around?"

"I became lost in composition, in the details of it. I became so wrapped up in finding the next note, the next sound, that the future couldn't touch me. I guess I started becoming numb to it, until it wasn't so scary anymore."

She nodded and looked away for several minutes. Finally, she spoke: "Promise me something: if you ever feel that way again, promise you'll talk to me, promise you'll tell me before you do something irreparable."

I looked deeply into her eyes: she was sincere.

"That's one hell of a promise," I said.

"Promise me!" she said angrily, her eyes flashing.

"Okay, okay, calm down. I promise." I returned to her side and put my arm around her. "It's all right. I'm fine now. The meds are working."

She smiled weakly.

"Listen, there is something else I wanted to talk to you about," I diverted. "Are you sure you want to go back to the States? Europe is much more conducive to the life we want. Classical musicians still have clout here. Just look at that family, how much they respected you. How many people in the U.S. take their children to classical concerts? More than half of the audiences here are young people. Back home, it's difficult to find a seat filled by anyone under sixty. The time when musicians like Bernstein rose to prominence, when the lines between classical and popular music became blurred, is long past. Guys like Bernstein and Previn were at the right place at the right time: the Jewish intelligentsia had recently fled Europe, and they were hungry for the culture they had left behind. Now, our people have become assimilated, as American as baseball. In fact, they'd rather watch baseball than Yiddish theater—or *any* theater. And where they go, so goes the culture of America . . . and it's going right into the toilet!"

"And so what then? Are we just supposed to stand by and let it happen, or—according to you—leave?" Dawn respond excitedly, beginning to pace. "Leave to come here? You said yourself that the Swiss made you feel unclean! Can you forget what they did during World War II—building underground weapon factories, laundering German assets so the Nazis could buy supplies? Once the rest of the world caught on to the Nazi regime, the Germans couldn't deal on their own, but they could through the Swiss. Without the cooperation of the Swiss, the war would have ended much sooner, and God knows how many Jewish lives would have been spared! And anyway, America needs people like us so they don't forget there is more to life than athletics—and money. The soul, the deeper emotions—the feminine in us— must be nurtured, too. Otherwise, society becomes more and more violent, until there is no society. Well, America is my home; I can't let that happen."

"And you're going to stop it, little ole you?" I asked with amusement.

"Yes!" she exclaimed passionately.

I walked over and put my hand on her neck, kissing her eyes, her nose. "I do love you . . . in fact, that's just what I wanted to talk to you about." I reached into my pocket and pulled out a tiny, black velvet box and snapped open the lid. Then, leaning on one knee, I grabbed her hand: "Would you make me the happiest man that ever lived by becoming my wife?"

Her face blanched so suddenly and completely that I thought she might faint. Then, she bit her lip, which was quivering. She looked at me for a moment that felt much longer, as the deep pools of her eyes began to overflow. Unable to speak, she simply nodded gently. Suddenly overtaken by emotion, I stood, grabbing her in a bear hug, squeezing tightly. I could feel her tears through my shirt, and I felt, more than heard, her words against my chest, near my heart: "Yes, with all my soul—yes!"

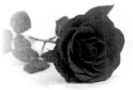

Atto II: THE BODY

The expression of the body of man or woman balks account,
The male is perfect and that of the female is perfect....
To be surrounded by beautiful curious breathing laughing flesh is enough ...
—Walt Whitman

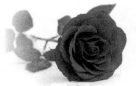

chapter 17: DAWN

June 1991

Tenerife: black sand beaches, sandy mountain ranges, camel safaris, topless sunbathers, and sublime Spanish brandy. What a place for a honeymoon! Our wedding had taken place in Baltimore, and Paul's parents had paid for this trip as a wedding present. I barely remember the flight: dealing with people, people, people at the reception had worn me out, so I slept through most of it. Sometimes, straining to follow the line of logic in a conversation or struggling to formulate the correct response felt like pushing a boulder up a mountain—with one hand tied behind my back. We had an afternoon reception so that we could make the standard evening flight to Europe. Nonetheless, we did not arrive in Tenerife until nearly the following evening, due to a long layover in London.

Then we endured an over-an-hour, bumpy, noisy bus trip to our hotel. The exotic scenery of palm trees and wild, unexplored mountains did not distract me from the fact that I was tired, hungry, overheated, and grumpy. My suitcase had been misplaced, so I could not even look forward to my own comfortable clothes. Despite the traveling, I felt more tired than I should be. After all, I was an experienced traveler; I should not be defeated by a no-pressure vacation across the ocean.

"When are we going to reach *our* hotel?" I snapped, after about the sixth stop, which was still not ours.

"It can't be much longer," Paul replied, reassuringly. "What's wrong?"

"I'm just tired."

The next thing that I remember was flopping head first into the soft whiteness of a queen-sized bed. I have no idea how long I slept.

I was awakened by the creaking of a door. It was Paul, returning to our room. When he noticed my opened eyes, peeking out from the covers, he said: "Tenerife is great! Do you want to get up and have a look around—maybe get something to eat?"

My body felt like an hourglass—a heavy, weighted-down feeling, moving from one part of my body to another. My head felt like it was wrapped in plastic. Yet, I did not want to disappoint my new husband, so I said: "Yeah, okay."

Well, Tenerife *was* great, but it was filled with many steep hills. The view of the ocean that Paul wanted to show me was at the top of one of the steepest. The nice thing was, there was a restaurant up there, too. Since I was feeling weak and could not see particularly well, the prospect of food was far more exciting than any view. I had noticed, recently, that I was no longer able to tolerate hunger. When I was younger, I was something of an ascetic and would go long periods without eating at all—sometimes, just for the effect, for the sense of control over my body. Perhaps I felt a need to punish myself, to become worthy of the talents bestowed upon me. My musical ability had garnered much attention from the age of five, yet I had done nothing to make this happen, nothing to deserve it. This had made me feel guilty, somehow. Too bad I hadn't been born Catholic: I certainly could relate to the whole guilt thing. However, in all seriousness, as fascinated as I had always been with the faith, it posed a few problems for me. For example, I could never figure out the point of purgatory. If God's grace superseded a person's good deeds, how could there be a middle ground? Either a person believed her sins were forgiven or she didn't. How could we "earn" a promotion to Heaven if all our "righteousness is but dirty rags"?

When I was very young, I also had a hard time with the contradiction of monotheism and the Trinity; however, as the Buddhist expansiveness that I had learned from my mother began to kick in, I realized that such a contradiction only proved the existence of God. I believed that there was one source, but that source had many facets, just as His reflection—the universe—had many facets.

From my father, I had assimilated the physical groundedness of Judaism: the love of family, the idea that one's earthly success is a sign of God's approval. However, this had always conflicted with my fascination for the ascetic, the monastic. I was, therefore, a contradiction all by myself. I could never figure out: how much of ourselves do we need to strip away to "get there" spiritually? If the physical world does not consume us, is it still a sin to love it? Perhaps it is only the more sensitive, the more impressionable among us that need asceticism. After all, some folks can be surrounded by the physical—money, sex, power, beautiful things—

and somehow never let it penetrate them. I was not one of those people.

Once in fifth grade, I decided to lose five pounds, just to see if I could do it. I restricted myself to one-half of a dry bagel for breakfast with a glass of water, nothing for lunch, and one spoonful of whatever stir-fry my mother happened to prepare for dinner, also with a glass of water. Five pounds quickly became ten pounds and counting, until my mother took me to the doctor. When the doctor told my mother that there was nothing wrong with me, my mother just sighed: "In Japan, after the war, I fought to get food, and now, in America, my daughter fights to avoid it."

Now, I felt like I could fight to get food. When I needed to eat, my thinking became muddy and my breathing, shallow. I was also having a lot of problems with my eyes. Sometimes, everything would just be blurry or I would see double images. Well, that was bad enough, but it was nothing compared with the times when objects seemed to leap into my space with no apparent warning. It reminded me of the message printed on a car's side mirror: *Objects appear closer than they are.* Oh, wait! I had that backward . . . *Objects are closer than they appear.* Images were continually flipping in my mind's eye. Yet, even that paled by comparison with the tunnel. I could be sitting quietly and, all of a sudden, my visual field would start to narrow, like someone was pinning blinders to the sides of my face. Then the blinders would become tighter and tighter, suffocating the light, until my world became surreal—and limited.

The restaurant was small and cozy, and the waiter was gracious. Paul ordered salmon, and I ordered the prawns. When our plates arrived, I was amazed, for I was accustomed to seeing prawns about the size of slightly bloated insects. These were about as long as my hand—including the fingers—and could almost pass for tiny lobsters.

I picked up one of the prawns, turning it so that its head faced Paul, maneuvering it like a puppet. In a high, cartoon voice, I asked: "Who are you calling a shrimp?"

"Wait!" Paul said excitedly. "I have to get a picture of this!"

"Well, hurry up! I'm hungry."

In one quick motion, he pulled out the camera and snapped the picture, saving for posterity the image of my holding the oxy-moronic sea bug.

"Now, *there's* an image for our children," I giggled. "Mama attacks unidentified sea creature!"

"And they'll probably ask: 'What's a sea creature?'" Paul mimicked a reedy little voice, then switching back to his own: "By the time our kids our old enough, there probably won't even be any sea creatures left—not the way we're polluting the waters."

"Bah-humbug!" I said, before making a sucking noise through my teeth. Without further ado, I peeled off the skin and bit into the prawn with relish. The meat was fishy in a good way and sweet, requiring no condiments of any kind.

We shared a banana flambé for dessert, taking turns feeding each other the syrupy soup. I had never done that before, and the experience was far more sensuous than I could have imagined.

Back at our room, there was a bottle of champagne, cour-tesy of Paul's boss, Maestro Kitajenko.

"Ah, that was very sweet of him," I said.

"Indeed—I'm quite surprised really." Paul covered the neck of the bottle with a linen napkin, like he was going to sever its head and couldn't bear to look the poor creature in the eyes. Gently, he moved the cork from side to side, popping the cork without popping it.

I smiled approvingly. "Nice. You know the proper way of opening a champagne bottle."

"Well, there's no need to make a big mess—besides, it's dangerous."

"I—hope you're that gentle popping . . . other things . . ."

His eyes filled with tenderness. "Don't worry."

The bubbles danced happily into our glasses as he poured, and we toasted *"L'chayim"*—"to life"—because we couldn't think of a more complete toast: when you have life, you have everything.

We took our glasses and went outside, on our small balcony. The salty air, the sound of the waves, and the shadowy moonlight against the dark mountains intoxicated us even before the champagne had a chance to kick in. I was beginning to come alive and although the misery in my body was still there, I felt capable of transcending it.

"Come here, you," Paul said playfully, as he cupped his arm around my back and pulled me toward him. My insides felt weak and tingly, simply from standing so closely to him. He kissed me gently at first, the soft skin of his lips brushing against mine. Then his mouth began to explore, his tongue softly prodding until I opened my mouth, which was all the incentive he needed to plunge his tongue inside. I was surprised by the intensity, and I moved back slightly while my hands grabbed his shoulders. His mouth traveled down my neck to the top of my breasts, and I began to feel a stirring energy deep in my abdomen. My long, flowing dress with low neckline gave him easy access, and before I knew it, he had unfastened my bra and had reached around to caress my breasts. My breasts were extremely responsive, as was his touch, which was fully tuned in to my reactions. Then his mouth took over, nibbling hungrily like I was the most delicious meal he had ever eaten. Pulling my dress below my shoulders, he found my nipple, which he sucked until I heard myself moan. "We should go inside," I whispered.

"I guess you're right," he mumbled, his mouth full of breast.

"Didn't your mama ever teach you not to talk with your mouth full?"

We departed from the balcony, but left the door open so we could hear the crashing of the waves.

We kneeled on the bed, facing one another, and I unbuttoned his shirt and slid my hand inside, feeling his strength, his hairiness . . . his manness.

As I caressed his chest, all of a sudden I noticed that I could no longer feel his hairs, his sinew. *Dear God, what is wrong with me?* Just like opening night in Bern, I could see my hand moving, but I could not feel what my eyes perceived I should feel. The realization frightened me, and I pulled back my hand with a start.

"What happened? Did I bite?" he asked with a perplexed look.

I shook my head. "It's nothing. It's just—excitement," I lied.

He grabbed my hand and began kissing each of my fingers. Although I could see this, I could not feel it.

We undressed one another and got under the covers, snuggling together. His hands began to caress every inch of my body, and I, his. Some of the touches—both received and given—I could feel; some, I could not. My heart began to race, and my vision darkened. I could feel wetness between my legs. Becoming lost in the sensations that I *could* feel was enough. My mind chased vision after vision, and yet I could not think. It seemed like we were falling into one another, becoming energy. My body was generating warm light that I needed to share. Three of his fingers clasped the nub above my wetness, moving in a slow circle. Like the hot wax of a candle after it has been run under a cool trickle of water, I had been melted only to become hardened. Clumsily, my hand groped to find him in the darkness. This time, I could feel, and the sticky hardness reminded me of a Popsicle. Perhaps this silly thought was my brain's attempt to distract me from the realization that, even though I could feel my hand again, I could not maneuver it the way I wanted. Nonetheless, the thought made me smile to myself.

"Ah, you like touching me," he said.

"Of course . . . why wouldn't I?"

"I just thought you might not—since, well, you have so little experience. Yet, that night in Vienna, I suspected you might."

"'I too am a continent / I have unexplored mountains, bushlands impenetrable and lost . . . No adventurer has claimed my desert valley's golden sands / Or crossed the virgin snows atop my highest barren lands.' Do you know Gertrud Kolmar's work?"

Paul didn't answer.

"Well, she was an obscure German-Jewish poet who died at Auschwitz before she hit fifty—and before anyone knew who she was. But more importantly, she was a woman who never married, never had a child. Yet, she wrote some of the most powerful portrayals of love and motherhood that have ever been written. My point is: a woman does not need to have experienced great passion in order to understand it."

"Okay, okay, point taken. Stop talking so much."

"I was just thinking we weren't talking enough. . . . Say something sweet to me."

"I love you."

"Why don't you use my name when you say it?" I teased.

"I love you, Dawn."

"That's it! That's all you've got! I thought you were an artist!"

"How about, you're beautiful."

"Ugh," I sighed. "Men!" I pulled my hand away and lay on my back.

"Women!" He mocked, as he resumed caressing my breasts. I closed my eyes to connect with his touch. Then I opened them to look at the man I had just married: he was perfect—slim but strong and muscular, hairy the way a man should be, and he had great hands. They were large but slender with long fingers—definite "piano hands." What's more, he knew how to use them.

"How about this," Paul started. "When I look at you with your eyes closed, I think: how could anything be more beautiful? Then you open your eyes, and I am lost!"

"You're full of it!"

"No—I mean it. It is almost too painful to gaze upon you. You are like the sun: beauty so intense it hurts. Memory does not do it justice. During all that time we didn't see each other— between Vienna and Bern—I imagined every inch of your face, your hands, every curve of your adorable body, but when I finally saw you in Bern, your beauty stunned me all over again."

"Hmm . . . that's good!"

"What I said or what I'm doing?"

"Both."

He pulled me closer. We couldn't seem to get close enough. I imagined the heat between us melting our bodies into one: *flesh of my flesh.* Would that be close enough?

He entered me slowly, and he felt nice going in, smooth and gentle. Then a sudden wave of pain engulfed me, and I bit my lip. It felt like I was being sliced into tiny little pieces. I heard myself moan—this time, not in a good way.

Paul remained perfectly still, except for his hand, which he brought around to stroke my face. "It's okay, sweetie . . . shush . . . I love you so."

We stayed that way for a few minutes, and then Paul moved ever so slightly. The pain was blinding. "Hon, you need to spread your legs more—you're so small," he said, with his hand on my right knee, pushing gently.

Deeper. Harder. For a moment, I felt objectified. Like a tight new shoe or glove, I needed to be broken in. Despite how much I loved him, despite the fusion of our bodies, I suddenly felt far away. My insides grew warm with bleeding, and Paul pulled out, turning to lie on his back. He put his arm around me, pulling me close. I nestled my face in the black curly hairs of his chest.

"I'm sorry, sweetie," he whispered. "It's always rough for a woman the first time. It gets better, I promise. That is, it will be better between us."

I reached down to stroke him, feeling my blood between us, feeling my blood uniting us. I was glad I had waited, glad I could give this man whom I loved every inch of not only my present and future, but also my past. I now understood why patience was such a virtue: it was not possible to find your soul mate, until you completed your own soul.

"Do you want to . . . climax?" I asked timorously.

He shook his head. "Not until I can bring you to climax. It won't be any good for me, otherwise." He turned his face toward mine. "And when I *do* climax, it will be to get you pregnant." He kissed me on the cheek.

"But, Paul, I went on the Pill last month."

He shot me an incredulous look. "You *what?*"

"I did it for us, in preparation for our wedding."

"But don't you—want a baby—with me?"

"Yes, of course, I do—more than anything. I'm just not ready . . . yet. Anyway, my endometriosis has been much worse. The Pill is supposed to help." I suddenly wondered what had made me think that, since the Pill hadn't helped the first time.

"I read somewhere that pregnancy helps, too."

"Hmm . . . that's always been the theory," I said skeptically. "I can't help wondering if that's just a variation of the same logic behind hysterical conversions—the poor, empty uterus causing misery throughout the body, pining for children. . . . Besides, how can I have a baby while on tour?" I had always believed I could do everything at once. Now, my body was making me believe differently. I didn't understand the source of this, and it terrified me.

"I guess you'd have to take some time off."

"But we need the money—especially now, with your going back to school."

"I still have my job at the symphony. I'm making the same money as I did before. Fortunately, in this case, less responsibility does not translate into less money. Besides, I'm resourceful: I'll find ways to get money. I always do. Don't kill yourself on the road just because of money. Now that you have your degree, you could even teach in a school system. If you want to tour, that's fine, but don't do it for the money."

"I love you—and we have plenty of time," I said, as I interlaced the fingers of my left hand with his. Our rings clinked together like wine glasses in a toast. Turning my hand to look at my rings, he said: "That is a lovely engagement ring, if I do say so myself. And I might add, simply seeing it on your finger makes me as rock-hard as that diamond."

Giggling, I groped for him with my free hand and replied: "Yes, it is a lovely ring. I love it! I'm glad they were able to size it down so nicely."

"Well, the jeweler laughed when I told him that you wore a size-four ring. He kept asking, 'Are you sure? Are you sure?'"

"I still don't understand why you bought it so large in the first place?"

"Well, I couldn't exactly have *asked* you what your ring size was, now could I? Besides, I figured that buying a ring was a lot like musical composition—as are so many things when you think about it. It's a lot easier to trim the excess than to put back what you've already destroyed."

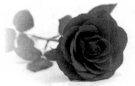

chapter 18: PAUL

January 1992

"Ah, I needed that," I exhaled as the heavy stein clunked against the dark wood of the bar.

"Yeah; you looked like you did," Xao said in his usual matter-of-fact tone. Few things got past Xao's shrewd eye. "You seemed distracted throughout the entire rehearsal. Is everything all right?"

I took another drink from my beer, trying to decide if I should tell Xao that everything was not all right. Xao was certainly one of the good guys: loyal husband and father, gifted musician, dedicated professional. He had been a violinist with the Bern Symphony ever since graduating from the conservatory eight years ago. He had been one of three exceptional students from Beijing who had been invited, as part of a cultural exchange between the two governments, to study in Switzerland. He was a cerebral player, with fine technique and precision. He was levelheaded, never late for rehearsals, and easy to work with—but he lacked spark. Perhaps, he was too level-headed—for a musician, at least. In this case, however, what I needed was levelheadedness. It was certainly in short supply these days. . . . Besides, I trusted him, both to be supportive and to keep a confidence. Nonetheless, the confidence was not only mine, it was Dawn's—in fact, it was even more hers—so I felt a bit guilty talking to anyone about it without her knowledge. Still, I needed to talk to someone.

"I'm—worried about Dawn. Her playing is not what it was." Now, why did I start with that? "I mean, she's forgetting more and more lately. And she's moody, irritable, and depressed. As a result, the intensity of our fights has increased. Have you noticed anything strange about her?"

"You mean stran*ger,*" Xao quipped.

"No, seriously!"

Xao shifted uneasily. "Look, I haven't really seen her that much since she signed with Columbia."

"Well, neither have I."

Xao smiled sardonically. "No, I guess you haven't. Of course, she acted pretty strangely at that rehearsal for the Prokofiev, but the actual performances were so spectacular . . . I don't know. Then, of course, when you told me what happened at the William Kapell Competition—how she made it to the finals, but was too weak to get out of bed the night of the final concert with the National Symphony. Dawn is way too ambitious to miss an opportunity like that unless she was quite sick, indeed. . . . And actually, though, there was something a bit more subtle. Remember at Hirsbrunner's dinner party, during that discussion on ethnomusicology when Hirsbrunner was recounting his extensive travels, and everyone was sitting on the edges of their seats—particularly when he talked about Egypt? Well, the conversation switched to a particular piece of music he had written and stayed there for more than twenty minutes. Out of the blue, Dawn asked the professor if he had ever been to Cairo. Well, earlier she had asked him specific questions about Cairo, and they had had quite a discussion. She seemed to have no recollection."

"Yes," I sighed. "I recall that incident. It was most unsettling."

"Well, it might not mean anything if it were an isolated occurrence, but I've repeatedly seen her interject questions or comments that are completely disjointed from the current conversation. Usually, I don't have the heart to redirect her. I have noticed that *you* don't hesitate to redirect her in front of others and—if you want me to be perfectly honest—that only makes her more self-conscious, and therefore, severely aggravates the problem."

"I know," I sighed, "but I become so aggravated. She's so intelligent, why does she do such stupid things?"

"I don't know, but they seem pretty harmless—though, of course, they are disconcerting. Like the one time I was over at your apartment, and she went into the kitchen to wash a dish, then flicked the light switch and just stood with the dish under the faucet, waiting for something to happen. She just stood there for a few moments looking confused, but then she figured it out and turned on the faucet. It's like her wires get crossed sometimes. She summed it up best herself. What did she say? 'That just reminded me of something—but I forgot what it was.' When she said that to me, in conversation once, I thought it was a joke. Later, I realized that she was quite serious."

"Well, I'm glad you have noticed, Xao," I said, with a heavy exhale, "because I thought perhaps I was going crazy—or crazier." I nodded to him with a smile, enjoying the private joke. "Since you have noticed, and you understand my concern, I'd like to share with you what has been going on. Our internist has referred us to many doctors, and they have tested her for everything from mono to a brain tumor. We've seen a neurologist, a rheumatologist, an endocrinologist, an infectious disease specialist, a cardiologist, and a psychiatrist—and those are just the ones I can remember after two beers."

"What have they found?"

"She doesn't have Epstein-Barr, thyroid disease, circulatory disease, arteriolosclerosis, diabetes, lupus, rheumatoid arthritis, an aneurism, or any of over two-hundred communicable diseases for which she's been tested. She's even been screened for bipolar disorder. So, basically, they haven't found a damned thing. And it's frustrating me to death."

"Well, just imagine what it is doing to Dawn."

"Yeah, I know. I'm being a selfish jerk, but I feel so helpless. I want to be able to *do* something to take away her suffering, but I can't. So, I just become angry. Sometimes, I even become angry at her—even though she's not the source of my anger at all. I'm angry at some outside threat, but she's there, so I rail at her. And because she's feeling bad, she's even more sensitive, and she cries. Then I feel guilty."

"Just remember, old man, that women cry for the same reasons we rail and cuss: it's just their way of processing the world, of releasing stress. It doesn't need to have any greater significance for them. It doesn't mean they are falling apart."

"Yeah, I guess you're right." I smiled as I took another swig of beer. Xao really did know something. "Except that she *is* falling apart in a way. Her hands hurt. She tries to hide it from me, but I can tell. She fights to practice through it, but she's practicing longer, with less effect. She can't get up in the morning. Some mornings, she wakes up with these blinding headaches. I've always been a morning person, and she's not; however, lately, she is taking it to the extreme. Now, most people return from tours exhausted, but she is beyond exhaustion.

"She also gets into more arguments with colleagues—more confrontations. She's become dogmatic about her decisions—you simply can't dislodge her. It's almost like she's afraid to step out of a groove, out of a pattern she's created. For example, in the Mozart 19—you know after the long *tutti*—she consistently comes in early. She never did that before, and she now insists she is doing it correctly. She also enters *fortissimo* and—you know the piece—the piano's entrance needs to be softer, more playful. Nonetheless, she insists her new way is correct."

"Did you ever stop to think; maybe she can't control the dynamics because she can't feel her hands?"

I was stunned. "Gosh, Xao, I *have* been an insensitive jerk! Why didn't I figure that out?"

"You're her husband—you're too close; of course, you are not going to see that. She's been invincible, and now she's not. Of course, you can't see that—you love her. Give yourself a break, man." Xao flagged the bartender, signaling another round.

"So, I'm not a jerk?"

"No, you're not a jerk. . . . Neurologist, huh? Sounds like the right idea. After all, for whatever reason, there have been a lot of great musicians—pianists in particular—with neurological problems: Gary Graffman, Byron Janis, Leon Fleischer. Nobody notices it until, well, it's there—whatever *it* is. I mean, until the symptoms become big. Look, I'm no doctor. I don't know what I'm talking about, but Dawn's problems certainly seem neurological to me. What did the neurologist say?"

I grimaced before speaking. "Are you ready for this? He was the worst. He just talked to us for about fifteen minutes, ordered no tests, and made Dawn fill out this ridiculous cognitive evaluation with questions like 'What day of the week is it?' and 'What kind of building are you in right now?' If she couldn't pass that, she wouldn't be cognitively impaired, she'd be practically comatose. Then he made her repeat a few simple phrases like 'No ifs, ands, or buts.' He barely examined her, except to put these metal instruments that looked like tuning forks on different parts of her body to listen for—something. Then he asked her how old she had been when she started playing the piano and how many hours a day she practiced."

"What does that have to do with anything?"

"Essentially, he was trying to make the case that all her symptoms were stress-related. In fact, he told her that she had put too many demands on her body, and it was calling out for a different kind of life. Can you believe that quack, putting all her symptoms down to overwork? I wanted to punch him out, right then and there!"

"I'll bet Dawn wasn't too happy about that either," Xao smiled knowingly.

I snickered. "Are you kidding? She was furious. She said to him: 'Oh, I suppose if I just stay home, clean the house, and raise children, all my problems will go away? If I were a man, you'd never tell me to give up my work! You'd look for a real disease!'"

Xao burst out laughing. "Did she really say that? Good for her!"

"Gee, Xao, I didn't know you were that liberated."

"I'm not, but you have to admit, she does have a point. That neurologist probably would not have treated either you or me that way. He would have at least run some tests on us. But maybe you should go back to the States and see some doctors over there."

"You know, you said that maybe she couldn't control the dynamics because her hands were numb, but maybe she played that way because her hands hurt—or both. Is that possible? God, maybe we should go back to America."

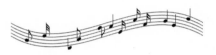

The walk home cleared my mind. The January air was cold and by the time I reached our small apartment, I had lost my buzz. The apartment seemed even colder than the outside—more from dormancy than from lack of heat. After all, I had been gone for over twelve hours, and Dawn had been gone for over three weeks, on tour in the States. I missed her presence, which brought softness to the dark edges of this Spartan apartment. We had confined ourselves to the basics: a worn, comfy old couch, a coffee table with more than a few nicks, a small dining table with only three chairs, a wooden rocking chair, a stereo, a small desk, a dilapidated console piano, and piles of books and sheet music— some in shelves, some in boxes, some just strewn about the room. Our bedroom was even simpler with only a bed, one dresser, another small desk—and more books.

Just as I had removed my coat, the phone rang. I picked up the receiver.

"Mr. Bailiff?"

"Yes?"

The voice on the other end proceeded to tell me that my wife had collapsed in the middle of her performance in Houston, Texas and had been taken to SCCI Hospital Houston Central.

When I hung up the telephone, I remembered that she was playing the Saint-Saëns Second.

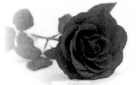

chapter 19: DAWN

January 1992
earlier, that same evening

I was sitting in the Spindletop Restaurant of the Hyatt Regency Houston, across from my former Peabody classmate and friend, Amy Hagaman, who was now first-chair flautist with the Houston Symphony. Built upon the rooftop of the hotel, the restaurant revolved slowly to give diners a bird's-eye view of the vibrant, modern city. We were sharing a pre-performance supper of pasta primavera, and being strangely hungry, I had far more interest in the meal than in the view. In fact, I had eaten two pieces of bread before our food even arrived. I never used to do that. It seemed that now I was always hungry, always eating, and yet I kept losing weight.

"Tonight's program has a few rough spots, doesn't it?" I asked.

Amy sighed. "Now that's a loaded question. What are you really asking me . . . or trying to tell me?"

Yep. This was the Amy I remembered: a real cut-to-the-chase straight shooter. Both her manner and her appearance were down-to-earth. She was your typical Midwestern farm girl who just happened to have a passion for classical flute, not to mention a singular talent which had taken her halfway across the country to Peabody. She was short—at 5'3" she was a few inches taller than I—and slightly overweight by societal standards but in an attractive, feminine way. Her hair was blonde and mousey, but her fair complexion was stunning.

Even though I knew it was probably pointless, I evaded her direct hit. "What makes you think I am trying to tell you something?"

"Oh, I don't know, little things like all through rehearsal you seemed distracted and irritable, and you've been flinching every time someone speaks to you—even our waiter just now. Besides, you're a results-oriented person: it's unusual for you to ask someone to dinner the way you asked me without a reason. . . . And your hands are shaking."

I quickly looked down at my hands: sure enough they were moving ever so slightly—definitely shaking. I quickly moved them to my lap, a maneuver that did not go unnoticed by Amy's sharp eye. "Okay, so what's *that* about?"

"Nothing."

"If it's nothing, why are you trying to hide it?"

I decided to turn the tables on her. "So, how's Margie?" Amy loved talking about her beautiful, two-year-old daughter.

"Oh, every day is a new adventure. You know what happened last week? I was getting ready to host a dinner party and had just cleaned my house from top to bottom. My nephew,

Christopher, who is four, whispered: 'Margie just told me she went poopie—in three different places.' Well, one-half hour before the guests arrived, my sister and I had to scour my pristine house, picking up my daughter's turds. Needless to say, they were everywhere but the bathroom."

We both laughed.

"And what about you, Ms. Newlywed, is Paul still pressuring you to have a child?"

"Actually, I had a miscarriage last month."

Amy looked both genuinely surprised and concerned, as she dropped her fork. "What? But the last time I spoke to you, you were on the Pill. . . . Gosh, I'm so sorry. That must be a devastating experience—I can't even imagine. So, that's it." She took a long swallow from her water glass.

"It is not *it,* exactly, though it's certainly part of it. And yes, I was on the Pill, but it affected me badly. I had to stop it." Reluctantly, I returned my hands to the table to continue eating.

Amy nodded. "Tell me about it! Weight gain, bloating, lethargy, depression. I even developed acne, which I never had before. I thought to myself, 'Okay, this makes no sense. I am taking this pill to have better sex and now, how am I supposed to turn on my husband if I am fat, pimply, and crying all the time?' Not to mention that it completely took away my sex drive. So, I stopped. That's when I became pregnant with Margie—but I don't regret it." She quickly held up her hand, lest I thought otherwise. "No way—she's the best thing that ever happened to me. I know women are always saying that, but it's the truth! . . . Oh, I'm sorry. That was stupid of me to say—I mean, in light of what you just told me." She lowered her gaze.

"It's okay. I wasn't even going there, so don't worry." I reached for my water, but I did not feel the glass in my hand.

Suddenly, it was no longer *in* my hand, but lying sideways on the table. "I'm so sorry; I'm such a klutz away from the piano!" I reached for my napkin to dab the water.

Assisting in the cleanup with her own napkin, Amy turned the glass upright again and said: "Ahh, don't worry about it. It's nothing."

"But anyway," I continued, after setting my wet napkin beside the empty glass, "the Pill didn't do those things you mentioned to me—except maybe the lethargy, but I'm always so tired that it's hard to tell. Actually, it was much worse; it gave me PMS. I didn't even realize what it was because I never had it before I tried the Pill a few years ago for my endometriosis. You remember—that surgery that forced me to miss all that time in sophomore year and led to my taking a break from Peabody?"

She nodded. "However, I thought you left Peabody to put some distance between you and Paul."

I smiled at her keen perception. "Well, yes, I did in a way, but that's beside the point. Anyway, for more than a week before my period, I became dark, clingy, paranoid, argumentative, and hypersensitive. I had a complete personality change: I perceived insults that were not there, and I felt more depressed than I ever thought possible. In fact, I had this sick joke with myself: as soon as I feel like cutting my wrists, it must be time to bleed. Paul was actually the one who noticed the connection between my craziness and the Pill. I just thought I was going crazy. The only thing I can say is that, while on the Pill, I just bled as opposed to hemorrhage—but what a price to pay."

"That's horrible," Amy said in complete sympathy.

"Well, you wanna know the worst part? Even after I've stopped the Pill, the PMS hasn't gone away. I guess I'm just stuck with it. It's tough to think about."

"Oh, gosh! That is depressing! What we women have to endure! Do you remember that birth control pill for men that they tried a few years ago but never fully released to the general public because of the side effects? Well, what could they be—a beer gut, hair in the nose, or a hostile temper? Like many guys aren't prone to those things already!"

Again, we laughed. It felt good to laugh: it had been a while.

"In all seriousness," I offered, "after experiencing them firsthand, I can't imagine that the side effects of the male pill could have been any worse than those of the female pill. So, it is unfair."

"Now, let's get back to you!" Amy persisted.

Gosh, she's relentless, I thought. As far as I knew, I had simply asked her to dinner because I didn't feel like being alone—unusual for me, to be sure, but not necessarily driven by some ulterior motive to bare my soul.

Besides, what should I tell her? Should I tell her that I had trouble seeing, thinking, and feeling, that I had bruises all over my body from falling for no apparent reason, that I wet my pants without even knowing I needed to go the bathroom? Should I tell her about the lengthy round of doctor visits, winding a long and rocky path to nowhere? Should I tell her about the far-fetched theories that ranged from potassium deficiency to hysterical conversions to depression? Should I tell her that the medical profession did not seem to take me seriously, calling my symptoms either stress-related or psychogenic? And worst of all, should I reveal to her my biggest fear: that Paul would begin to believe them?

How could I tell her about the night before I had left to go on tour, when the distance between Paul and me had been so vast, I would have needed an ocean liner to cross it?

We had been drinking champagne on the roof of our apartment building. It had begun to snow, and the snowflakes had landed in our glasses, keeping the wine chilled. I had marveled at the magic of this: tiny, little snowflakes falling from the sky, ending their lives as sugary specks, doing a final dance amidst the bubbles in my drink before I swallowed them, merging myself with the heavens. Unfortunately, at that moment, I had lost connection with my hand, flinging half of our wine glass collection to the hard rooftop, splattering champagne and glass shards all over Paul. One runaway sliver had actually cut him right below his eye. All of this had happened shortly after I had forgotten about an important development at the *universität* that Paul had supposedly told me a few hours previously. A development that, even now, I could not remember . . .

"Paul, please don't pull away from me," I had pleaded. "I am so, so sorry about all of this . . . but I am not doing it on purpose!"

"I know," he had replied distantly, "but I don't know what else to do. I feel so helpless. I don't know what you need."

"Just love me," I had responded.

"I already do. Once, I thought that was enough . . . I guess it's not."

That night, I had initiated sex for the first time. I had been too terrified to admit to my husband—even more terrified to admit to myself—that I could not feel him inside of me. . . .

"Hey! Are you listening?" Amy said loudly.

"I'm sorry—what?"

"I *said:* you obviously didn't take much time off for the miscarriage. Are you okay?"

I shrugged. "I don't know. Work helps. However, this tour has been particularly brutal, but I only have one more city to play after Houston. Then I can go home, which is a good thing. I'm really tired."

"But what happened?"

"They don't really know. I was having a lot of pain in my lower back. One night, I went to bed, and the pain became so intense, there was nothing else. I must have bled so quickly and severely that I passed out because I don't remember any of it. Paul told me that he had been awakened by my moans to find me, literally, in a pool of blood. The only thing that I remember is waking up in the hospital, with Paul sitting on the bed and the doctor standing alongside. These two men told me that *we* had lost the baby."

"Talk about unfair," Amy commiserated.

"Well, I don't know about that, exactly, but it just felt strange. I mean, I had just gone through this horrible ordeal—this completely female ordeal—and somehow, these two men had claimed it, somehow they owned it. I still don't know what to make of it."

"I understand," she reached out to squeeze my hand.

"The strange thing is that being pregnant actually improved all the really weird symptoms, but since the miscarriage, they've become much worse." Oops! I let the cat out of the bag this time, for sure.

"What really weird symptoms?"

"Oh, nothing really," I back-pedaled. "Just extreme tired-ness—and some shakiness." I did not want to shine the light upon this monster; I just wanted to shove it into the closet and lock the door.

Amy nodded skeptically. "Uh-huh. Okay, Ms. Immovable Feast for Man's Senses, be that way. But if you don't talk to me, you're gonna have to talk to someone."

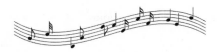

I felt a certain kinship to conductor William Henry Curry. Born in Pittsburgh, he began his conducting career at age fourteen. Like me, he came from a blue-collar town and began performing seriously at an early age. He was also a member of a minority.

Bill Curry became resident conductor with the New Orleans Symphony in 1990, and he was juggling his responsibilities there with a series of five performances of Leroy Jenkins's opera, *The Mother of Three Sons,* at the Houston Opera from October 1991 through the upcoming spring. Tonight, he was guest conductor for the Houston Symphony.

He and I also had history. He had conducted the Peabody Orchestra and had been resident conductor of the Baltimore Symphony Orchestra from 1978 to 1983. I had soloed for him and the BSO at the age of thirteen, playing the Tchaikovsky Piano Concerto no. 1, and again the next season, playing the Saint-Saëns Piano Concerto no. 2—the same piece I would be playing tonight.

I had played with the Houston Symphony several times before, under music director Sergiu Commissiona. The first time—at age eleven—had been part of an eight-city tour. And I had worked with Maestro Commissiona before that; the first time had been in my hometown when he conducted the BSO. Ah, the music industry: what a small, small world. . . .

The backstage lights at Jones Hall seem harsh as I wait to perform one of my not-so-favorite concerti. The piece is a bit too schizophrenic: the first movement is nearly suicidal, while the final two movements are spirited and jovial—too weird, even for me. Nonetheless, I learned it nearly ten years ago because Curry had requested it. And I am playing it again, tonight, for the same reason.

I give the keys of the Baldwin Concert Grand a final good-luck stroke before it is wheeled onstage. I watch it almost like one watches a good friend going to the gas chamber, knowing that she, herself, will be close behind.

I don't feel right. Hands feel particularly numb. Shake out my hands in an attempt to regain feeling. Mind-numbing headache. A strange sensation in my left forearm, like insects crawling down my radius bone. Feels like my hands have been severed at my wrists—or like there is a band, cutting off the blood supply to my fingers. My sight is distorted: cloudy and painful. Sounds seem hollow and slower. I am scared, but I still have to perform tonight. Again, I shake out my hands. My brain feels like it's been packaged in cellophane. My life force feels compromised.

Curry approaches me and shakes my hand. "Good to see you," he whispers, stepping aside to allow me to walk ahead of him. My journey down the dark corridor seems surreal: I hear the sounds of the audience, alternating between loud and soft, fading in and out. In one moment, I can hear the details of the most private conversation, and in the next, all I can hear is a whir. *Well, despite the 800 adjustable hexagons constructed into the ceiling to regulate the sound, the acoustics in this hall have always been unclear,* I assure myself.

I step onto the stage, feeling cocooned within the stage lights. Again, public privacy. Curry, who has followed me onstage, grabs my hand, and we bow together to the sound of the applause. Then we turn and nod to the orchestra. I go directly to the piano and miss the bench, nearly falling before I manage to sit.

G minor. The piano has a long solo in the beginning, which almost sounds like a duet—the bass and the treble banter back and forth like a man and a woman. The woman wants to fly and the man protests, trying to keep her grounded. Finally, they merge in a resistant passion, which is predominately feminine. And the struggle continues into a series of somber bass chords: big, bossy, and dogmatic. When the orchestra comes in, it sounds a little like Mozart's Requiem Mass, but this quickly relinquishes to a romantic melody, lushly dark, foreboding, then nostalgic. The music is too painful—it separates me from myself. At least, I think it is the music that is doing this. Glassy couplets in the high register make me feel that I am dying, suddenly connecting me to the beginning and the end at the same time: babies in their mothers' arms, old people breathing their last breaths, and me, disintegrating into vapor, becoming nonexistent—everything that I was, evaporating. I am beyond all thoughts except one: I miss my life, yet I long to be more because my life is closing in. My brain turns inward on itself, so that I can see myself dying. I am both afraid and unafraid, breathing and resisting breath. My humanity rails in self-defense, in desperate crashing passage-work that encompasses the entire keyboard. The numbness in my hands switches to stabbing pain. Then, I feel numbness and pain simultaneously. I do not understand this, but I am split between my sensation and my self. I can actually sense the signals that my brain is sending to my hands. They are moving so slowly, I can feel them traveling down the nerve pathways, struggling to reach my hands. I have to concentrate to make my hands respond: there is no automatic response. The effort is immense, and it takes everything I have—every ounce of power still remaining in my body. My brain seems to disconnect, but I cannot feel what it is disconnecting from. I am separated from myself, but I am still aware that my self exists. Yet, I cannot find it. . . . pounding, percussive . . . suddenly, the entire left side of my body disappears. I cannot feel my leg, my foot, my arm, face, torso—nothing. In my left eye, there is only darkness. It is difficult to breath, and my sense of being becomes distorted. *Dear God, am I having a stroke? Is this it?*

I fall off the bench. I am flat on my back in front of over 2,000 pairs of eyes. The stage lights are too penetrating for my one remaining eye. Too bright. Then, somehow, I know it's over. The music has stopped. At least, for me.

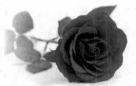

chapter 20: DAWN

January 1992
that same evening, continued

I awakened at Houston Central to someone jabbing my right forearm with a needle and saying something—rather loudly—about blood gases. "We need to get to your artery, okay? This is going to hurt a bit—more than a blood test—but it won't last long."

A bit? My muscle began to contract, and it felt like the early stages of a menstrual period were taking place inside my arm. "Why didn't you use my *left* arm," I groaned with difficulty. "I can't feel anything there . . ."

My headache was so bad it was more like head *pain*. The pain was jagged and pressing, pushing out any possibility of rational thought. Every time I tried to move my head, I had to wince. My hair felt heavy against my skull, and there was a stabbing pain in my right eye. My left eye felt like it had been jabbed out by a hot poker: there was only strange heat and blindness.

The pain in my head seemed to make my arm hurt—or was it the blood gas thing? Or did my brain distort my perception of the blood gas thing? Did it even happen? I figured I had better check.

"Why did you do that?" I asked the woman with the needle.

"To check the oxygen in your blood, which tells us the condition of your lungs," she said. "The card in your wallet said you have asthma, and you have a Proventil inhaler in your purse. The overuse of short-term inhalers can sometimes cause fainting and numbness—even temporary paralysis."

Overuse? "I haven't used my inhaler in ages," I said. I had even forgotten it was still in my purse.

"Okay, fine. I'll make a note," she said curtly. There was a loud rustle as she left. Or was that my roommate turning the pages of the *Houston Chronicle?* I turned my head to look at her, wincing as I did so. Evidently, my supposed good eye was not working correctly either, for the woman in the neighboring bed looked like a two-dimensional shadow, emanating green light.

"Do you have the Arts section there?" I asked.

"I'm sure I do," the shadow replied.

"Could you read the review of last night's symphony concert to me?" At least, I thought it was last night.

Again, the rustle. It traveled up my spine like a chill. "Guest conductor Maestro William Curry gave the citizens of Houston a stellar performance . . ." The words began to blur together, but I just kept listening for the word *piano.* "An engaging conductor—both verbally and musically."

"Is that it?" I asked.

"That's all of it," the shadow replied.

"Thank you," I said slowly. All that effort had worn me out. *Cowards,* I thought, as I faded into sleep. But I was glad they hadn't mentioned me . . . glad, for once, to be invisible. . . .

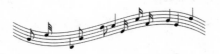

I had been in the hospital for over two weeks, during which time I had more tests than I could even begin to recall. I had been rolled into long tubes to allow penetrating looks at my insides, connected to wires, injected with dyes, electrocuted with probes, pierced in the spine with needles. For a woman who had spent her life holding conventional medicine at arm's length, I had certainly been getting one massive force-feeding to make up for it. I had never felt so helpless and so degraded in my entire life.

Finally, one morning, the doctor in charge of *project moi*—who had barely said three words to me in the past week—stood next to my bed, peering sternly at my chart.

"What time will your husband be here this evening?" he asked without taking his eyes off the chart. "I need to speak to both of you."

"He should be here about six," I replied.

"All right. Fine. I will return after six."

And that was that. I had the entire day to do nothing but lie in bed and wonder what news the doctor had to convey that was so terrible, he just wanted to say it once. Then I became angry: as a woman, did my body command so little respect that its welfare was of greater significance to my husband than to me? Yet, I was simply too weak to expend much energy dwelling on this issue—and even less on trying to change it.

I could not move anything on my left side. I felt split in two, caught between feeling and unfeeling, like there was a border strip traveling down the center of my body, dividing what still existed from what did not. And what existed was pain. Spidery fingers of pain sprung from the top of my head and crawled down the right side of my face, extending their jagged, pointy nails deeply inside of me.

There was a ragged heaviness in my right arm, which felt granular. It migrated up and down, moving when I moved like sand in an hourglass. Again, the hourglass.

Pools of throbbing overflowed into rivers of splintered ice. Sharp edges that penetrated like arrows took turns radiating from every inch of my right side: eye, eyebrow, jaw, neck, chest, forearm, elbow, wrist, palm, fingers, fingertips, hip, thigh, calf, foot, toes . . . I had never before been so aware of all the different intersections and bumps in the winding path of my body. Before, it had seemed like one smooth, uninterrupted stream, flowing quietly without detour.

My left eye was still completely blind, but I was now able to make out the features of those around me. I could not tell if this was due to an actual improvement in my right eye or to an adjustment made by my other senses.

At 7:00 p.m., my husband sat on the edge of my bed with his hand resting on my right knee, while Dr. Wizard sat some distance away on a high-backed, wheeled chair.

Dr. Wizard spoke: "Judging primarily from the extensive lesions in your wife's—ehr, in *your*—brain and spinal chord, as evidenced by the MRI, *and* the abnormalities observed in the spinal fluid, my colleagues and I feel confident that a definite diagnosis is in order. We believe multiple sclerosis is the culprit."

I felt Paul's hand stiffen upon my knee. He looked at me very quickly, then back to the doctor. "But doesn't that put people in wheelchairs? What is it exactly?"

Thus spake Dr. Wizard: "MS is a disease of the central nervous system—constituted by the brain and spinal chord. Nerve fibers within these organs are protected by a membrane called myelin, which functions much in the same way as does insulation on an electrical wire; that is, to keep impulses flowing smoothly from point *A* to point *B*. For reasons we do not yet understand, in multiple sclerosis, the body looks upon its own myelin as foreign matter and attacks it, replacing it with scar tissue, hence *sclerosis*. This interferes with the transmission of nerve impulses and eventually destroys the nerves themselves. The upshot: bodily functions become uncontrolled. The way this manifests varies greatly from person to person, and even within an individual's experience of the disease. Some folks *do* end up in wheelchairs, as you pointed out; many others function quite well with the use of a cane, brace, or crutches. Some folks need no assistive device at all. As I said, the range of symptoms is wide. Most MSers do experience extreme fatigue, pain, numbness, lack of coordination, difficulty walking, slurred speech, dizziness, heat sensitivity, headaches, tremors, and intermittent blindness or blurry, distorted vision. Optic neuritis—inflammation of the optic nerve, cognitive difficulties, and loss of bladder and bowel control are also common. Paralysis may occur, as may damage to the nerve pathways that control involuntary functions, such as breathing, heart rhythms, hormone production, and digestion. You should know as well . . ." he suddenly lowered his voice and spoke even more directly to Paul than he already had, ". . . that sexual problems also occur. . . . I am sure you understand."

I was too humiliated to speak.

Paul assumed his take-charge stance. "Well, what do we do? How do we cure it?"

Suddenly, I found my voice. I knew a thing or two about MS—my first cousin had been battling it for nine years. "There is no cure. Is there?" I asked flatly, staring coldly, mercilessly at Dr. Wizard.

He met my gaze for a moment, then looked away nervously, all too quickly, as he spoke: "No. There is no cure."

Paul simply could not get his mind around this. "But, what do we *do?* Why now?"

Dr. Wizard again: "Judging from the lesions, it is my suspicion that your wife has probably had MS for several years now. This is not unusual: many patients have the disease for years before noticing symptoms. It typically strikes in the prime of life—between the ages of twenty and forty—and affects well over two million people worldwide, 350,000 in the United States alone. It affects more women than men—the ratio is 2.6 to 1—so there is probably a hormonal component. . . . Although pregnancy sometimes triggers a remission of symptoms, childbirth, itself, is hard on the disease. Many women experience an intense flare-up of their MS within six months of giving birth. We don't entirely understand it—but we do know it has something to do with hormonal fluctuations. Nothing is more hormonally traumatic than a miscarriage: one minute the body is pregnant, the next it is not. Your wife's miscarriage probably triggered this intense flare-up.

"Of course, there is no way of knowing this with absolute certainty." He paused a moment for this to sink in. "As for what we can do: there is a new drug in clinical trials that will, in all likelihood, be approved next year. It is an interferon; the brand name is Betaseron. Many doctors feel it holds great promise; however, its effects on the disease are not yet conclusive. And there are some pretty nasty side effects."

"But wait, you said that won't be on the market for another year—what can we do *now?*" Paul persisted.

Dr. Wizard nodded once in acknowledgement. "You could attempt to get into a clinical trial. However, we can treat flare-ups such as this with intravenous steroids a lot more quickly and effectively. We administered an emergency dose when she first arrived, following up with prednisone, which seems to have been quite effective in taking her out of critical mode. When she arrived, her breathing and metabolic functions were severely compromised. . . . This is what I would advise right now: a more formal course of IV steroids, keeping a careful eye on the situation. We don't yet know what the course of her illness will be. Judging from the severity of this attack—and the extensive nature of the lesions—I suspect we are dealing with a particularly virulent type, most likely a progressive form. Again, I suggest for now, we get her out of this intense flare-up. Then we sit tight and see what develops."

Even in my confused, weakened state something about this did not sit well with me. I deeply resented the way that, contrary to holistic practices, traditional medicine persisted in divorcing the patient from her self, from her own body awareness. But I looked over at Paul, and he seemed satisfied. Clearly, I was outnumbered. I was still too numb from the news of my diagnosis—the full impact had not even begun to take hold. Besides, as much as I mistrusted conventional medicine, the prospect of fighting *for* "nasty side effects" did not seem like a viable use of my limited energy. So, I went with the program.

As it turned out, the steroids had plenty of nasty side effects of their own—including bloating, nervousness, heart palpitations, and good old nausea. Nonetheless, I was glad I was actually beginning to feel well enough to be cognizant of these side effects. *Oh, well,* I thought. *This will all be over in a few more days. This flare-up will subside, I'll go home, and everything will be back to normal.*

Ah, yes, ignorance is bliss. At that time I had little knowledge of what lay ahead:

Flowers:
These pangs of color are like feelings,
painted faces intermingling
within each other's roots. Their
unadulterated flare
in death reminds me
I too am strong.

I await the doctor's verdict.
"What time will your husband be here this evening?" he asked with icy eyes, frozen
to my hospital chart. "I would prefer to speak with both of you."

That was 9:00 a.m. It is noon, now. My fear has hollowed me out, and I am raw.
I have another 6 hours to live with unknowing,
before the spotlight traps this elusive Monster that has pinned me to the bed.

Although we have not yet been formally introduced, I first became acquainted
with His huge claw,
as it sideswiped my left eye without warning, leaving me in chiseled darkness. Frequently,
He seizes my hand and won't let go, until I drop the pen, the book, the glass . . .
Sometimes, for fun, He kicks my leg from underneath me, and He likes to make me
doubt my ability
to speak,
to think,

to swallow—
just in case I happen to forget He's there.

He has come between us, though I did not invite Him. I wonder if His name will make
a difference.
I fight to reach through His gnarled body, lest you forget: I am still here.

Funny how gentle flowers do not depict gentle feelings—I've always wondered
what delicate, dying plants have in common with the powerful eternity of pain,
death, or even, love.

Please do not bury the edges of my eternity searching for rose petals.

Your attempts to absorb my pain only give it wings, passing the poison back and forth;
my guilt singes me slowly, and I feel my identity shrinking
like the wick of a candle.
I do not want to hurt you by dying.

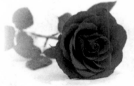

chapter 21: PAUL

June 1992

I finished reading the poem Dawn had left on my desk. The poem was entitled "Flowers" and used the roses I had sent to her in the hospital as a metaphor for her feelings about her diagnosis—and also her feelings about *me,* surrounding her diagnosis. The poem was painful to read, but I was grateful for the insights it gave me. Since she had returned home to Bern three months ago from the Houston Institute of Rehabilitation and Research, she had been writing vehemently. And that was not all she had been doing. I had to admit that I was amazed how well she was coming along, all things considered. Although I had not originally approved of the natural course she had decided to take, I had supported her decision. And now, there was no denying that it seemed to be working for her. Nonetheless, I was still worried. After all, in her weakened state, she was naturally vulnerable to all the radical, new people she was encountering on her journey: she had had a difficult time, and the difficulties were far from over.

After a month in the hospital, Dawn had spent six weeks in the rehab center, receiving physical, cognitive, and occupational therapy, as well as basic care. I still felt terrible about having to leave her there in Houston all that time, but what else could I have done? With the sudden loss of income from her concerts, it became imperative that I continue to earn a living, and my work was here in Bern. Someone had to pay for all this, and that someone certainly couldn't be Dawn. I had also been in the final throes of my doctorate—which, thank God, I just completed—and I just couldn't have thrown that away. In a field as competitive as ours, I needed that degree to open more doors—especially now, the freedom to remain in one place, teaching at the university level and/or doing research was a freedom I could not afford to lose.

Besides, the long trip would have been brutal on her, and even if she could have made it home, her condition at that time would have required some type of nursing or assistive care during my working hours. We simply could not have afforded that and would have had little chance of receiving assistance as foreigners in the convoluted, socialized structure of Swiss medicine. So there it was: I really had no choice . . . but that fact did not assuage my guilt.

So, I did everything I could. I kept busy researching clinical trials and MS specialists, and installing bars in the shower and ramps over the wooden room dividers in our flat.

When she had first come home, Dawn had been in a wheel-chair, but recently she graduated to crutches and a brace on her left leg. She was still quite fatigued, so she tired easily. She also had bouts of extreme dizziness and frequent falls. But this was, still, so much better than she had been. The vision in her left eye had returned, and, overall, she seemed to be thinking better—although we certainly had our moments. For one thing, her monthly hormonal fluctuations had become much worse. This increased her dark moods and, therefore, our arguments. I couldn't help thinking that this was some sort of poetic justice: now I was getting a taste of what I must seem like to others without lithium.

One evening, about a week after she had returned home, I was working at my desk, which was the one in our bedroom. She wheeled in behind me and, for a moment, just sat there, staring. She had a glass of red wine in the little caddy I had rigged to her wheelchair to hold beverages. As she stared, she picked up the glass, shakily, and brought it to her lips. Then, in an instant, she poured what was left in the glass down my back, forming a red river on my white dress shirt from my neck to my belt.

I sat up with a start, reaching to the back of my neck to feel the wetness, to check if what I perceived had really occurred. "Damn it! Why did you do that? What's wrong with you?" I shouted.

She replied tearfully: "Why won't you talk to me?"

"I have no idea what *you're* talking about," I said hotly.

"Ever since I've come home, you've been cold and distant. You've never even kissed me! Aren't you glad to see me? Don't you still love me?"

Now, that was insulting; I became really angry. "What kind of craziness is that? Didn't I practically redo the apartment so you could get around? Aren't I doing all the shopping and cooking besides working my job and going to school? I worry about you night and day—what do you think?"

"You don't have to do all the cooking," she said softly.

What could I say? I knew she enjoyed cooking and wanted to reclaim her turf. I had resisted because her hands were still so unsteady and her ability to multi-task was so impaired that she found it difficult to ensure that all components of a meal came together at the same time. As a result, her recent efforts in the kitchen had only left me with more work. I suddenly realized how unimportant all that really was.

"I just want to be close—the way we were," she continued. "I miss you. I'm still the same person. I can still feel."

"Can you?" Now, why did I say that?

She flashed me a look of pain. "Yes, I can—in *here.*" She pressed her knuckles against her heart. "The body is only a shell, you know? It's only a tool."

"But how else can I get to you?" I asked desperately. "Without your body, you won't be here. Without your body, you'll be . . ." Suddenly, I found myself choking back the tears. I was surprised and embarrassed. I turned away.

Her hand grabbed my wrist. "Don't hide your fear from me . . . don't!"

"Don't *you* do this to me—don't make me face the prospect of losing you!"

"But you haven't lost me: I'm here! Don't treat me like I'm already dead."

Ouch! She got me: that's exactly what I had been doing. I was so afraid of losing her that I had already begun to pull back, to distance myself. But she was still here, she still needed me, and most importantly, she still loved me. And I still loved her. But I was afraid to touch her. Yet, there was no way of avoiding risk, even without the love we shared, *especially* without the love we shared. . . . What a fool I had been.

Nonetheless, Dawn did not make it easy. After I had found a clinical trial and had taken considerable pains to have her considered, she refused to follow through, saying that she would not pollute her body with "further toxins." She started playing with crystals and magnets and asked me to buy her meditation tapes. A few of them, including *Creative Visualization* by Shakti Gawain and *Self Healing* by Louise L. Hay, actually seemed to help her. In fact, I think those two tapes had a lot to do with her getting out of the chair. She made an intense study of Buddhism, sitting zazen once a week with a group of people from our apartment house. I actually did not mind that so much because, after all, she was half-Japanese, but what really bothered me was her relationship with the woman who lived directly above us. Nicole was originally from Quebec and was a born-again Christian. She took Dawn to a few services where people actually talked in tongues and collapsed on the floor from the power of the Holy Spirit. She gave Dawn a copy of the New Testament to read—in English. Dawn seemed quite interested and read it often. This gave me an uneasy feeling, but I did marvel at Dawn's voracity—and persistence—in reading. Although the vision in her left eye had returned, she still had myriad visual disturbances, including blurred vision, impaired color and depth perception, eye fatigue, and pain.

Overall, her pain was what most concerned me. Although she tried to hide it, I knew her too well for the deception to succeed. I could not always discern the source of her pain—the endometriosis or the MS—but I knew, in either case, it was severe. Sometimes, her body seemed guarded, tight, like it was all she could do to keep herself protected from the monster. The problem was that the monster came from the inside. Her threshold of pain humbled me, for her only pain medication was an occasional glass of wine. Unfortunately, the wine seemed to aggravate her PMS.

Late one night, during her first month back and around that time in her cycle, I returned home from a concert to find her sitting at her desk—which was the one in our living room—crying over a big, thick book. When I asked her what was wrong, she flipped furiously through the pages and began reading in a shaky voice: "'The pastoral images of contented animals grazing in the barnyard are a thing of the past. Today, a chicken may never see a speck of real sunlight from birth to slaughter. Raised in cages too small to allow free movement, they get no exercise. In fact, their food, laden with chemicals, antibiotics, and hormones, is brought to them on a conveyor belt, and their wastes are removed in the same way. As a result, they often become too big for their legs to support them and, if they did have room to move, would need to slide on their breasts.'"

"What is that?" I asked.

"Just a book on modern farming practices . . . listen to this: 'Steers are taken from their mothers almost immediately after birth and fed powdered milk, laced with antibiotics and other medications. Later, they are fed processed food that includes not only antibiotics, but also growth-enhancing hormones. When the steer reaches six months, it is placed in a pen with twenty-four-hour artificial lighting to alter sleep patterns and encourage continuous eating of not only grains and synthetic carbohydrates, but also shredded newspaper, plastic pellets, and recycled manure. After four months of this, the steer, weighing over 1,000 pounds, receives a few more doses of antibiotics and hormones as a pretenderizer and is sent to slaughter.'" She looked up from the book with tears streaming down her face.

"I can't believe that," I said. "That's too terrible—what kind of propaganda is that?"

"It's *not* propaganda," she protested, rummaging through a pile of papers and pulling out a small pamphlet, which she waved in the air, then opened to read. "This is from documented sources. Now, listen to this: 'Of the 143 drugs and pesticides identified as likely to leave residues in raw meat and poultry, 42 are known to cause or are suspected of causing cancer, 20 of causing birth defects, and 6 of causing mutations.' That's from the United States General Accounting Office!"

"Where did you get all this stuff?"

"In Houston. The Institute's library was fantastic. I spent a lot of time alone . . ."

I looked away.

"I *mean* it provided an excellent opportunity," she added quickly. "Look, this is serious, and it's just the tip of the iceberg. Our fruits and vegetables are loaded with pesticides; much of our food is genetically mutated or at least processed into something completely different from what nature intended. I mean, for Pete's sake, take white bread, for example: they actually remove the most nutritious parts of the wheat—the bran and the germ—bleach what's left with chlorine gas, and dump synthetic versions of the very nutrients they just removed back in! What kind of egotistical craziness is that? Do we really think we can come up with a more perfect food source than the natural plants themselves? And look at milk: did you know that when they first started shooting cows up with synthetic hormones, forcing them to produce more milk—artificially and against their natural, female cycles—some of the farmers actually noticed that their wives and daughters developed menstrual problems after drinking this milk? Can you believe that this didn't even stop them?

"Can't they see, we are all God's creation, we're all one? You can't destroy one part without destroying the whole. Well, the cows are my sisters, too. They give live birth and nurse their young. I'll bet they're capable of getting PMS, too, and they probably feel really awful on all those hormones. I can't condone that happening to another female—even if she's a different species."

"Well, what are we supposed to do about all this?" I asked, numbly, still stunned by the tirade.

"Buy organic. Perhaps, don't buy meat at all."

"Well, I'm not giving up meat. . . . Tofu is for wimps. Besides, it's disgusting—it makes me think of *Soylent Green.*"

"But they are killing us with all this garbage! We are even becoming more vulnerable to various strains of infections, thanks to all the antibiotics we're ingesting! This European diet, with all its meats and rich sauces, is killing us, and you're too blind to see it!"

"Well . . . I'm not giving up meat."

"Then maybe you should take up hunting."

"What?" I shook my head and began walking toward the bedroom. I was glad she was taking an interest in something again, but I was more than a little concerned for her sanity. "The only thing I can say is that they must have given you some really good drugs at the rehab center."

She ignored this comment and plowed on. "Oh, come on, you like guns. Don't you think you'd find it relaxing?"

"Oh, please! Remember when we visited those Italian friends of Xao's, and I couldn't even look at that cow's head, sitting on the coffee table? All those other people were picking at it like it was a plate of chips and dip, but I had to leave the room—remember? Some hunter I'd make!"

"Well, if you can't commune with the animal who gave his or her life for you, if you can't face the reality of where your meat comes from, maybe you shouldn't eat it. Just think; you're swallowing all that denial, all that fear, and internalizing it. It's dishonest. It's no different than a woman wanting to have a baby and getting knocked out for the actual birth."

I shook my head and laughed. Perhaps I should be annoyed, but this entire conversation was just too bizarre.

"No, I'm serious! I remember reading that a lot of rich women in the '50s used to actually *request* a C-section, even when there was no medical reason for it. I think Jackie O was one of them. Anyway, talk about fear and disconnection. It's like they were saying, 'Oh, I'm too prim and proper to spread my legs and have this baby rip its way out of me on its own time. That's only for peasants!'"

"Perhaps."

"In any event, diet is the key to health—and this Northern European diet has too much fat, too much dairy, and not enough vegetables or whole grains. It is toxic, and there is a lot of evidence that toxicity is a factor in MS. For example, MS was first described in 1868 by Jean-Martin Charcot in Paris—*1868*. That was around the Industrial Revolution, when the use of chemicals in everything we eat, touch, and wear became widespread! Nonetheless, I think I've come up with a solution: Zen macrobiotics."

"Macra-what?"

"Macro-biotics. It is the diet used in the Zen Buddhist monasteries. It would be a great way for me to reconnect with my heritage."

"Your heritage is Ashkenazi, too. The best way for you to reconnect to your heritage through food would be to throw together a tofu and matzo sandwich!"

"Oh, hah-hah—actually, I have done that! But seriously, in the monasteries, this diet is referred to as *Syozin Ryori,* which basically means 'cooking that promotes supreme judgment.' Essentially, the body is like a bank: you can't take out what you don't first put in. Anything we do that violates the natural order of the universe will trigger disease. Western medicine is goal oriented: 'Find a cure, find a cure.' But they are wrong. The goal is not to find a cure—to win—for that only promotes stress. The goal is to find balance."

"Between what?"

"Us and the universe, with the Tao—with nature's way. I was wrong to be so competitive in my music, so hungry for success. True, I started out just loving my art, wanting to produce something beautiful, but it all became twisted—twisted by greedy people wanting to sell my talent, to turn me into a product, a plastic thing, no longer myself, just a better model of everyone else. And I let them do it, and it almost killed me!"

I walked over to her, pulled her wheelchair from behind the desk, and turned her toward me. Then I leaned down and kissed her. "Sweetie, I really don't think you contracted MS as a punishment for being ambitious or eating slaughtered animals."

"That's not what I'm saying."

"Sure it is—I know what's really behind all of this, my little ball of guilt."

She sighed and looked down at the floor for a few moments. Then she spoke more quietly: "Would you do something for me?"

"You mean besides grabbing a rifle and combing the Berner Oberland for our dinner?"

She smiled. "Yes, *besides* that. Could you check the university library to see if they have a copy of *Zen Macrobiotics* by Georges Ohsawa?" . . .

Well, I did find a copy of the book—in French. It was an amusing scene: my half-Japanese, half-German–Jewish wife, cooking Japanese food from a book written in French by a Japanese man. Talk about the long way around.

In time—although she never talked me into eating tofu—I actually developed a taste for the whole-grain rice, colorful roots, mushrooms, and even the seaweed. I must confess that as a result I developed more energy and clarity of mind.

Besides, that episode was nothing compared with the next month.

Despite the downright pathetic condition of her hands, Dawn practiced piano continually, throughout the day and evening; she practiced through her pain, her frozen fingers, her disconnects. And the music she produced was painful—both to hear and to watch. Her fingers slipped, along with her memory: she would hit sharps instead of naturals, naturals instead of flats. She would begin the cadenza of the Beethoven *Emperor Concerto* only to switch to the first movement of the Brahm's Piano Concerto no. 2 after playing only three lines. Sometimes, her hand would simply flop from one chord to the next or freeze up in mid-phrase. The pain in her body was obvious: her back was tight, her brows, tightly knit. Often, she bit her lip. Occasionally, her hand flopped backward like a desperate fish, and she cried out in pain. The really sad part: the more she practiced, the worse she played.

At first, I let her do her thing, for I knew how difficult it must be for her to lose her music. Whenever I tried to put myself in her place, imagining what it would be like never to conduct again, I was unable to think beyond the initial shock. Truly, I had no idea how I would survive or even if I *could* survive. So, I tried to give her room. However, there came a time when I just could not take it anymore. She was living in the past and that would be of no help to her or me. As long as she persisted in trying to regain what she could no longer have, she could never be free. And because I loved her, neither could I. Besides, she was torturing herself and although it was noble, it was unnecessary . . . and unfruitful.

One evening, her playing was particularly awful, and I was particularly tired. To listen to this woman who was once so masterful make so many mistakes was just too much, and even though I knew she was hormonal and that I should probably restrain myself, I just couldn't.

I set the textbook I had been studying on the coffee table and looked at her. "Why don't you give it a rest?" I asked as gently as I could.

"I have to—get it back . . . it will come back . . . I *know* it will! I just have to push through the pain. I can't give in! The pain doesn't matter; only the music matters. . . ."

"Remember what the latest neurologist told you? MS is not something you can just 'push through.' Overexertion only makes it worse. If you push too hard, you'll push yourself right into another attack. Do you really want to get to the place where you can *never* hold your own wineglass or a fork?"

"But I can do it—I know I can!" She kept playing—or trying to play.

In desperation, I walked over to the piano and placed my fingers on one of the knobs, sticking out of the keyboard protector. "Move your hands, please," I said. "Come on, lights out!" I began tugging at the lid. Begrudgingly, she moved her hands and sighed loudly as I pulled the wooden cover over the keys. Furiously, she wheeled away, practically running me over.

"Damn it! Don't treat me like a china doll, like I'll break or something!"

"Then stop trying to break yourself."

"Well, I *am* going back to school next year, whether you approve or not," she snapped, out of the blue. "I have to do something besides wheel around this apartment, while you stand vigil, waiting for me to drop dead!"

Without telling me, Dawn had applied to a special dual master's program in Educational Philosophy and Technical Translation between German and English at the University of Vienna. The program was specifically geared to artists and those with undergraduate degrees in an artistic discipline who wanted to become teachers or scholars of Rudolf Steiner's philosophy. Essentially, Steiner believed that the arts could be the vehicle to teach any subject and that the cultivation of independent free-thinkers was education's highest goal.

Dawn had been accepted into the program, which meant she would start this fall, which meant she would need to move to Vienna. As crazy as I thought the whole thing was, I knew she needed to try. But there was no way I was letting her go to Vienna by herself.

"And what will you do if you get really sick again, all by yourself? How will you take care of yourself? How will you get around? Vienna is not exactly handicapped-accessible."

"It's only for nine months. Besides, I'll be out of the wheelchair by September," she said flatly.

"And what if you're not?"

"I *will* be."

"But what if you're not?"

"Then I'll figure it out by doing it!" she snapped. "Do you think this *thing* is stronger than I am?" She slapped her palm against the plastic arm rest. "Do you think this chair will stand in my way? Well, it's just a tool, a means to an end—no more or less than my body, itself!"

I placed my hands on either side of her, clutching the armrests of her chair, so I could lean my face in close to hers. "You talk tough. Well, I know you're tough, but don't be a fool. What are you going to do if you need to get in or out of somewhere with a flight of stairs and no ramp or elevator? What are you going to do—rely on the kindness of strangers—strangers who will take advantage of you, who might rape or kill you for a hundred schilling? What will you do when you can't feel your money in your hand or, worse yet, can't even see it? How will you wheel yourself down cobblestone streets or access stores and restaurants that are separated from the street by even three or four narrow steps? What if you have a memory lapse and can't remember where you wrote down your address? Let's face it: your days of traipsing around the world alone are over—get used to it!"

"Oh, I see *now* what I look like to you! I see!" She choked as she lowered her eyes. Then she froze in shock. "Oh, I didn't feel it. . . . I didn't know." There was a puddle of urine below her feet. "Sometimes, it just comes out all by itself—without my feeling anything," she said quietly.

"See what I mean?" I asked just as quietly.

Flashing me a hurt look, she grabbed a dish towel from the back of a dining room chair and began dabbing her dress, her legs. "You think this proves anything? You think this means I need to be kept under lock and key? Well, I'll show you! I'm going out—alone!"

"What—like that?"

"It's just urine—urine is completely clean when it leaves the body . . . especially if you drink plenty of water, and you're not toxic," she said as she threw the dish towel on the table. "I'm going out, in this chair, just like this—and don't you *dare* try to stop me!"

"Yeah, great! Fine! Do whatever you want!" I said in exasperation. Although I was worried sick, I was pretty fed up. Besides, this was not New York—or Baltimore; it was Bern: you couldn't find much safer streets. And so, she wheeled out without even so much as grabbing a sweater, leaving me to chew my fingernails for the next three hours.

Nonetheless, it was worth it, for when she returned, she seemed transformed:

"Well, I hope you are satisfied," I said in a wounded tone. "I was worried sick."

She motioned for me to lean closely to her and when I did so, she gave me a passionate kiss. "I'm sorry about that," she said, "but I needed to make a point. You have to give me some room. You have to trust that I learned something about my body through all this."

I nodded. "So what's that?"

"A book. This man at Zither's Inn gave it to me." She held up the book that had been wedged between her right thigh and the side of the chair so I could read the multi-shaded pink cover, obviously designed by Peter Max: *Survival into the 21st Century* by Viktoras Kulvinskas. I took the thick book from her hands and quickly thumbed through the pages: it was wild.

"Wheat grass juice? Colonic Irrigations? Aquarian Liquid Diet? Help me out here!" I pleaded for understanding.

"As I said, there was this man who helped me up the steps," she said, averting her eyes. "Well, I knew right away he was

American—an expatriate, like us—anyway, we struck up a conversation, and he asked me why I'm in the chair, so I told him."

"Just like that?" I asked incredulously.

"Just like that. *Any*way, he tells me that he is a survivor of tes-
ticular cancer and that he owes it all to this book. I ask him where
I can find such a book, and he tells me that he carries an entire
case of them in his car for occasions just like this one. Then he
goes out to his car to get a copy and gives it to me, free of charge!
I mean, the guy's a regular Pied Piper for Viktoras Kulvinskas.
The work saved his life, and he feels it is his duty to the universe
to share the wisdom. Isn't that wonderful?"

"Hmm."

"He also gave me the names of several resources," she continued, fumbling around in her pocket. "One of them is a natur-
opath here in Bern by the name of Dr. Bloch. The other is in the
U.S., in Virginia Beach, it's an acronym . . . oh, here it is." She
handed the paper to me.

"A.R.E.?"

"Association for Research and Enlightenment. It's devoted
to the work of Edgar Cayce—you know, *the* man, when it comes
to modern holistic medicine. This guy figured it all out!
According to Doug—that's the man I met tonight—by the way,
he's invited us for dinner—well, Cayce actually devised an entire
protocol for curing MS naturally. We have to send for it tomorrow!"

"Yeah, okay—whatever. So tell me about this guy, Doug.
What did he want exactly?"

"I'm telling you, he didn't want anything. He's just a guy
who has been through a lot, and he knows something—and he
wants to share that. That's it. That's all there was to it."

I wasn't so sure, but at least I was convinced that was all there was to it for her. And that was enough.

"Okay, so what's the point of all this?" I asked.

"In a nutshell: to detoxify the body so it has the strength to tap into its own natural healing resources, to work *with*—not against—the natural order of the universe. . . . Look, the macrobiotic diet is a good start, but it might not be enough. I think I need to speed up the process, to thoroughly detoxify my body, and this book shows me how. Wheat grass is key. We can even learn to grow our own."

"But where do we get it?"

"That's where Dr. Bloch comes in. Besides, the detoxification process is a bit rough; we might need some help. . . ."

Well, she was right about that. We did see Dr. Bloch, and Dawn did start a detoxification regime, using wheat grass juice, organic fruits and vegetables, and Mu tea. On the second day, she developed severe cramps and a high fever. On the third day, she began throwing up, and her heart rate accelerated, hitting 120 beats per minute. By the fifth day, her fever had broken and was replaced by cold, trembling sweats. Naturally, by this time, I was quite concerned, so I took her to see Dr. Bloch. He told us this was all pretty normal, but he administered intravenous vitamin C and glutathione—which the body, itself, manufactures to detoxify the liver—to speed up the process. He also taught us how to make a supportive tea, made from blackberry, celery, chaparral, goldenseal, and rosemary. Dawn was to drink the tea three times a day.

"Also very important," he said, "is to take a detox bath. You must wash yourself thoroughly first. Then draw a bath as hot as you can stand without it burning you, adding one-fourth of a cup of Epsom salts. Then you must shower thoroughly afterward. This is important."

"But that's a problem," Dawn said. "MS patients cannot tolerate heat! In fact, one of the first tests for MS was to immerse someone in a hot bath. If she became fatigued or developed other neurological symptoms as a result, she was diagnosed with MS."

"Then you must start slowly—five minutes the first day, seven minutes the second day, and so on, until you can sit comfortably for thirty minutes. Increase the Epsom salts gradually as well, by one-fourth cup a day, until you reach two cups."

"What do Epsom salts do?" I asked.

"The sulfur pulls environmental toxins from the body," said Dr. Bloch. "It also increases blood supply and alters the pH of the skin. This is very important. Much disease stems from an imbalance in the acid-alkaline ratio. Too much acid creates inflammation, which is linked to many disease processes. The skin is really just one big porous shield between the body and the outside world. If the skin is in balance, it will effectively thwart the assimilation of further toxins.

"After you become accustomed to the thirty-minute bath with two cups of Epsom salts, replace the salts with a cup of brewed blessed thistle tea. Again, it is most important that you take a shower immediately after you bathe; otherwise, your skin will simply reabsorb the toxins."

Dawn turned to me: "Wow, with my mobility issues, that's going to be a lot of work. Even with the bars in the shower, I'll need your help . . . do you mind?"

"Any excuse to put my hands all over your naked body," I ribbed.

All in all, the detox took about two weeks. Afterwards, Dawn was so weak, it was difficult to tell if it had actually done any good. To rebuild after the ordeal, Dr. Bloch prescribed some-thing called Km Liquid, of which she worked up to two teaspoons a day, along with Sun Chlorella, of which she eventually took six tablets a day. To help the kidneys do their job, he had her boil a bundle of parsley for thirty minutes and drink the resultant fluid three times a day. Gradually, she did seem stronger and more clearheaded, but her mobility had not improved. By then the Cayce protocol had arrived, and we were hopeful. The protocol came with a wet cell battery with a solution of gold chloride, which needed to be used every day for thirty minutes to promote nervous system rejuvenation, followed by a massage. Cayce believed that the system's inability to assimilate gold was at the root of the problem, for he saw gold as a key nutrient to neuro-logical health. His theory of the pathology behind MS was simple: the nervous system is vulnerable to the efficacy of the overall cleansing mechanism of the body. Just like any other bodily sys-tem, it requires good nutrition coming in and toxic wastes going out. Specifically, he felt that MS stemmed from a failure of the glands, particularly those associated with the liver, to produce the substances necessary to maintain neurological health. Since Cayce put much weight in the spiritual attitude of the patient, viewing the glands as the body's link to the soul, one's glands could not function properly if he were spiritually out of sync—nor could he develop spiritually if his glands were compromised by toxicity.

Although I was still skeptical about all of this, I knew Dawn was committed to it, and as long as she was committing to life in some way, that's all I cared about. Besides, I had to admit that something was definitely going on within her body. Exactly what, however, I was not sure.

While going over the Cayce protocol, we made an interest-ing discovery: the protocol was not contradictory to anything we had already done; in fact, it only reinforced it. Cayce stressed how important detoxification was in MS and alluded to poisons produced by the nervous system that may destroy myelin.

The diet that he suggested—fruits, vegetables, and fish, with a reduction of fat and the elimination of processed foods—was in keeping with the macrobiotic diet. In addition, the Zen macrobiotic focus on "the way" (from the Greek: "macro" meaning "great" or "comprehensive," and "biotic" meaning "way of life") as opposed to the cure was directly aligned to Cayce's belief that the patient's attitude should be: "The physical conditions that have come upon me are those most necessary for my own soul's development" (Cayce readings, 716-1).

Nonetheless, with all of this, Dawn's progress was far from dramatic. "In the end it all boils down to the spirit," she sighed dejectedly. "And I am still so spiritually confused. Cayce talks about patience, how the only way for one to truly learn her own soul is to develop patience, but I have no patience. For me, waiting has always been the hardest thing of all."

"I think you're selling yourself short," I replied. "It takes great patience to practice an instrument for six hours every day for nearly twenty years. Don't confuse a lack of patience with drive."

"Okay, but what about 'applied spirituality'? I don't even understand what that means. How can I do it?"

"It will come," I reassured her, like I knew something. In reality, I had no idea either.

The entire process seemed to totally absorb us, bringing us closer together on some level, but binding us into a cerebral, obligatory routine on another.

It did not help matters that her numbness and reduced sensation transferred over to the bedroom. Sometimes she had difficulty maintaining arousal, which led to even more pain than her endometriosis already caused. However, I had an idea.

"I have a surprise for you, but first you have to sit over here," I said, setting a plain brown box on the bed.

"Okay." She held out her arms for help, and I scooped her out of the chair and sat her upon the patchwork quilt she had made in high school—the one she had saved for her first child.

She opened the box and pulled out a hand-sized appliance with provocative attachments.

"What do you—do with it?" she asked timorously.

"What do you think?"

"But how does it work?"

"Why don't we find out?" I attached a rubber piece that looked like a thumb and forefinger held in the shape of an "L," like someone imitating a handgun, and flipped the switch. The vibrator made a steady whirring sound.

"Uh, that's loud," she said.

"I'm sure we'll get used to it." I started at her right calf and moved slowly up her leg, circling her inner thigh. "Do you feel that?"

"Hmm . . . yes . . . keep going."

I moved the vibrations to her abdomen, again circling slowly. Then, working under her dress, I followed the line of her breastbone to the area between her breasts. She wasn't wearing a bra. Her nipples were hard. I started to pull her dress over her head, and she helped me, giggling slightly. As I leaned down to suck her breast, I moved the vibrator between her legs. She moaned slightly, reaching to unzip my trousers, putting her hand inside. As far as I was concerned, she still had great hands. With some difficulty, she wriggled out of her panties.

"You have the greatest ass," I mumbled against her breast. "And I still love your smell." Again, she giggled.

"I love yours, too."

I leaned the rubber attachment against her, brushing the outside of my fingers against her wetness. She tried to pull me closer, but our little mechanical friend got in the way. I set it down, so I could touch her . . . so I could feel flesh against flesh. Grabbing hold of my belt, she pulled me toward her. Moving against me, she tried to unbuckle my belt, but the task was too intricate for her hands. She bit her lip nervously. Gently, I removed her hand and did it myself: "It's okay," I whispered.

By now, she was attempting to unbutton my shirt, but her fingers stuck and fumbled. There was pain in her eyes, then tears. "I'm sorry," she said. "I'm so useless."

"Don't be silly," I reassured her. "Just go back to what you *were* doing with your hands." She smiled softly.

I found our friend, and we tried again. When I could feel her wetness dripping on my fingers, I inserted the rubber forefinger inside her and rested the faux thumb against her clitoris. I moved my hand slowly back and forth, but I didn't have to do much: the machine did most of the work. Watching her move was a real turn-on.

I couldn't believe the power of her hand: she had enveloped me in her touch, which knew my body so well, I could want nothing else.

"I'd rather have your hand than another woman's vagina," I whispered.

She studied me with her eyes; then she sniffled.

"What's wrong?"

"Nothing. I'm so happy. I love you so."

"I love you, too."

She groaned in pleasure as she climaxed against me. I could feel her left hand trembling against my back. I came almost immediately afterward, releasing myself into her hand, falling limp against her. . . .

Later, she looked the vibrator over carefully, studying its contours. "You know, this might work really well when we . . . that is, we could try . . . I mean, maybe if we just use the tip and hold it off to the side, at an angle . . . it might work *while* you're inside of me."

"I think they have smaller gadgets for that purpose," I replied. "But it's worth a try."

"Hmm . . . After all, you're not the one who has difficulty multi-tasking. . . . Somehow, I don't think this is what Cayce had in mind when he referred to vibratory medicine."

Even climaxing was hard on her neurology: she was always more numb, confused, dizzy, and generally unsteady for as much as a day afterward. Sometimes, her headaches even became worse. I guess that's not so hard to understand when you think about it: having an orgasm is a pretty intense physiological process that involves much of the nervous system.

So, it was difficult, but I tried. We both tried. I knew that her desire to please me was sincere, and in the final analysis, that's the sexiest thing there is. She always had some book around with a goofy title like *How to Please Your Man* or *How to Bring Your Man to Ecstasy in 10 Minutes or Less.* I remembered coming home one night to a bathtub full of lime Jell-O. She said she wanted to try making love in it because she had read about it in *The Sensuous Woman.* Well, why not? She was trying—and it was different, no doubt about that. And it *was* fun . . . even if I did have lime Jell-O coming out of every orifice for the next three days.

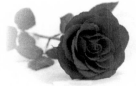

Atto III: THE SOUL

Be not ashamed women ...
You are the gates of the body and you are
the gates of the soul.
—Walt Whitman

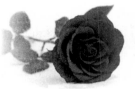

chapter 22: DAWN

July 1993

Ocean. Mountains. Blue sky. White vapors giving the illusion of substance. I had always loved flying. This flight reminded me of my first time: I had flown, with my mother to Chiba, Japan, to visit my grandparents, as a small child. Coasting down the runway, accumulating speed, gathering momentum felt very much the same as practicing the piano: I would start out slowly, timidly, even resistant. But as soon as my fingers made contact, I was off. The hardest part was getting started: cranking the motor. *A body at rest remains at rest; a body in motion remains in motion.* If I allow myself to stop, what will become of me?

After I was married, I realized that the actual ascent into the air was a lot like sex: tension building, movement increasing, adrenaline pumping until the anticipation was simply too much and then . . . using the physical surface to springboard into . . . something else. That something else was, in turn, a lot like the mystical transcendence I was struggling to attain—or maybe, it *was* the mystical transcendence: using the body as a springboard into the soul.

I had always been tuned in to energies I did not understand. As a child, I could communicate with my sister telepathically, and I had always been able to see different colors—which I later learned were auras—around people, animals, and sometimes even objects, if they held particular meaning for a living being. In addition, going out of body had seemed to come naturally to me. However, music had always been my primary connection to other-worldliness, my passport to the divine. I knew of nothing more perfect than sound channeling feeling. Music was a way to get to the back of the mind, to go beyond the mind, to become fully alive without concrete thought. The only other entity that came even close to this on the physical plane was love.

Three days ago, we drove to Geneva to spend a few days there before flying to Seattle, Washington. The flight from Geneva, Switzerland, to the U.S. West Coast was fourteen hours long, and despite my love of the experience of flying, the change in atmospherics and air quality was hard on my MS, turning the whole thing into something of an ordeal—yet another thing MS had taken from me. All the flights from Switzerland to Seattle left from either Geneva or Zurich—not from Bern—so we drove the slightly less than one-hundred-mile trip from the home we were leaving behind. Besides, we had already rented a car to get to Bern, and we needed a breather between the flurry of moving out and the chaos of moving in. Although we had been living in Vienna for the past ten months, we just closed on the sale of our Bern apartment and had numerous details to settle before leaving the European continent—probably for good. At least we had been able to spend a little time with Xao and his family and a few of our other Bern friends, whom we hadn't seen much of since moving to Vienna—such as Doug and his wife, Joyce.

On the way to Geneva my period hit, and by the time we had settled in for the night, my endometriosis was in high gear. The pain, as usual at that time, was difficult to endure. Despite our sometimes bitter arguments over the preceding few days—due to the intensity of my PMS, coupled with the added stress of the move—Paul was wonderfully sweet to me, making me tea, rubbing my back, holding my hand. The pain was so bad that his hand upon my lower back made me wince, but I was grateful for his touch.

Although our holistic efforts had improved my MS—I had been walking with the assistance of two canes for one month short of an entire year!—attempts to find an effective pain remedy had eluded us. Both the valerian and cramp bark that Dr. Bloch had suggested worked on some level, but their effects on my neurology were terrifying. The valerian, in particular, caused me to have what I had named "disconnect attacks," which felt like my mind was being disconnected not only from my body but also from my soul. The weirdest part was that I was able to see the process happening in slow motion: I knew what was coming, but I could not stop it. The apex of these attacks was pure terror. It was as if a huge, impenetrable wall had been abruptly erected to separate me from myself. Many medications actually had this effect on me, including antihistamines, ibuprofen, the most powerful antibiotics, and narcotic pain medication—all of which I vehemently avoided. The only times I had experienced them were when they had been thrust upon me in the hospital.

A well-respected herbalist in Vienna reminded me that I must look at the pain from the perspective of my inner self as well as my outer self; therefore, the hormonal—the emotional—symptoms needed to be treated along with the pain. On the internal plane, he explained that there were two categories of PMS: the one that provokes tears and the one that provokes rage. Whichever category a woman fell into determined which herbs she should take.

I said: "Well, I'm in *both* categories, so what should I do?"

"I think, in your case, if you take care of the 'angry pain,' the tears will take care of themselves," he replied and proceeded to mix up a batch of *lung tanxieganwan*—a Chinese brew of numerous herbs, including ginseng. This purportedly worked by cleansing the liver and gallbladder—toxins yet again! Nonetheless, after several months, neither the anger—nor the pain—had improved.

I also tried dong quai, a Chinese herb that was said to be the female toner, balancing the hormones, reducing pain and bleeding. However, in my case, it caused hemorrhaging. Meanwhile, the herb, chaste tree, had no discernible effect on me at all. Raspberry leaf tea would reduce my bleeding, but since it stimulated uterine contractions, it also increased my pain. This seemed a cruel trade-off to me—and one I could not afford when I was already in so much pain. The effect was similar to that of the ergotrate, which the conventional doctors had given me after my miscarriage and on several other occasions when I had nearly bled to death from endometriosis gone awry. Ergotrate stopped the hemorrhaging, but it did so by increasing contractions of the uterus, which caused intense pain.

About the only concoction that offered acceptable relief was a cup of strong peppermint tea with a few dashes of cayenne pepper. Cayenne pepper was my saving grace; it instantly made me feel better. According to *The Healing Power of Herbs* by May

Bethel—one of the books I was reading on the plane—cayenne is "one of the strongest and purest stimulants known" and "the key to success in medicine is stimulation." Essentially, cayenne acts as a catalyst, heightening the body's natural healing powers.

Nonetheless, sometimes—like that first night in the Geneva pension—it was simply not enough. It was in those moments that I really learned to pray, ironically reverting to the prayers of my childhood, repeating the Shema Yisrael over and over:

> *Hear, O Israel: The Lord our God, the Lord is One!*—
> *And Thou shalt love the Lord thy God with all thy heart,*
> *and with all thy soul, and with all thy might....*

And that was it: right there. The alpha and the omega. There comes a point when you simply figure out there is nothing to figure out. In the "dark night of the soul" there is God—emptiness is not vacancy; it is part of God. Everything—which includes nothing—is part of God. On some level, I had always known this; perhaps, the acknowledgement of it had been my greatest fear.

For much of my life, I had struggled so hard to reach the unreachable. I had shaken the tree of dogma and ritual, hoping to dislodge even one piece of fruit that I could digest, that would not make me puke. I was beginning to learn that the rituals, the prayers, were simply tools—just as my body was: a springboard into . . . something else.

The underlying history is merely a distraction. What the prayers, the rituals, say to *me*, right now, to my mind beyond mind is all that matters. Supposedly wise men and women have studied entire lifetimes, only to return to this simple truth.

Lying in terrible pain on that strange bed in Geneva, clutching a large slab of amethyst that Doug had given me (in crystal therapy, amethyst is known to combat female pain), I suddenly stopped trying to rail against the pain. Instead, I dove directly into the middle of it—as I had my fear that night in Bern— becoming intimate with every splinter, every jagged edge. I discovered that I could do this, and I would not disappear, that there was still life on the other side. A strange power overtook me, and although the fear was still there, it no longer altered anything. I could feel the fear and the pain and sacrifice nothing. My body was big enough for all of us.

In that instant, all the knowledge I had accumulated over the past several years came together: the Asian focus on finding "the way" to self-realization instead of a "cure"; the holistic view that healing must take place on all levels—mind (attitude), body, and soul; the need to love and respect one's body by feeding it healthy, spiritually aligned food sources that do not compromise one's ethical code and by giving it room to eliminate its toxins and rejuvenate itself. Through all this I had learned that the greatest physician anyone can consult is oneself.

If you have faith, nothing shall be impossible to you. That was one of my favorite passages from the New Testament. But I did not need the New Testament for this: Buddhism, Judaism, and even metaphysics also stated it. And since we were created in God's image, we can't have faith in God without first having faith in ourselves.

I felt I had, at last, uncovered the key to Edgar Cayce's "applied spirituality"—my missing component of his MS protocol. In his readings, Cayce said that it was not only important to be good, but also to be "good for something." *Faith without works is dead.* Faith is a verb.

What doth the Lord require of thee? the prophet Micah asked. *Only to do justly and love mercy and walk humbly with thy God.*

"Walk humbly with thy God"—now there was a real koan, for true humility before God lay in the realization of self, of how powerful a being a human truly was. Perhaps that didn't make sense, but I had also learned that if an insight into the soul did not make sense, then that was probably because it did not make sense—and least not to the rational mind. And sometimes, it was okay not to make sense. Sometimes, it was only through not making sense that one could find true awareness, healing, or enlightenment. My readings of the mystical literature had taught me this—especially the books of the *Zohar*. And yet, independent of all these books, love had taught me this.

During my "dark night of the soul," after sitting with me through hours of intense pain in our rented room, Paul, at last, stepped through my thorny cage and scooped me up, becoming like a soft, big blanket, encasing me. He put me in the car and just drove—without destination, to the place where we no longer needed to make sense. We were traveling anywhere—nowhere—and there was only us. Us. And the darkness, and the headlights, and the motion, and the cold and the heat. We talked but said nothing. We wanted nothing. Nothing but to melt into the darkness and into each other. Nothing but to triumph over pain. . . .

I was deeply moved by the fact that not only had Paul decided not to thwart my efforts to study in Vienna, he had actually given up his position at the Bern Symphony and found one teaching conducting at Vienna's *Akademie für Musik,* so he could move to Vienna with me. It was wonderful to realize he respected me that much, that he valued what I was trying to do. I was particularly moved that—even after he had grown to detest the politics of his job and the fact that he was not actually permitted to teach anything real at all—he stuck it out until I received my master's.

During the past year, he had often spoken of his love for his hometown—Seattle—and how he longed to return. I agreed to move to Seattle if he found work. Due to the fact that his father, a highly respected professional—a veterinarian—in the Sea-Tac area, sat on many artistic committees and boards, Paul had less-than-average trouble securing work for the upcoming fall. Not only was he stepping in as principal conductor of the Tacoma Symphony—which was actually only a part-time position—he had also secured an assistant professorship in composition at the University of Washington.

In my own right, I had already completed the preliminary application process for a teaching job at the Seattle Waldorf School and was scheduled for a series of interviews the following week. I was fully confident that I would be offered a position. There was a sudden opening for the fall, which simply seemed synchronistic. . . .

The plane hit an air pocket, and I instinctively reached for my glass of wine to steady it. Wine: my one deliberate toxin. Or was it? Wine had certainly been with mankind since the beginning as a symbol of life, blood, prosperity, and reverence. Interestingly, despite alcohol's potentially damaging effects, my inner wisdom had guided me to it. When the pain was particularly intense or I was not in a position to find a quiet place to reside within my pain—like when crammed into the seat of this airplane, for example—a glass of wine worked quite well, filing down the most serrated edges of the pain. And as for my neurology, the pain seemed to absorb the alcohol like a big thirsty towel, leaving no excess to seep into my fibers or irritate my nervous system. As long as I drank only what I needed for pain, I felt no sense of intoxication.

I had also begun to look at wine differently since Paul and I had, in this past year, returned to our Jewish roots, not that we had ever denied being Jewish or stopped thinking of ourselves as Jewish—but we had given up the *practice* of Judaism. Even this, however, had not been a conscious decision; it had just happened.

Strange as it may seem, it took a study of Christianity—of the New Testament—to bring me back to Judaism.

Well, actually, I had been studying the Buddhist Sutras, looking for answers, when I met Nicole, our born-again upstairs neighbor. The services she took me to were uncomfortable at first: people chanting, yelling, speaking languages they had never studied. However, something intrigued me, compelled me to return. On my third visit, in a moment of prayer, I asked God to make his presence known to me; I invited him to enter my body. Then, I remained open. After a few moments, I felt a spiritual presence enter my body that was pure energy, pure love. For a few seconds, the presence lifted me to a new awareness: it was ecstatic. The best way that I can describe it is an orgasm of the soul. Then I heard myself mumbling words I did not understand: "Oh deus ay oom. Oh deus ay oom." Suddenly, my body went limp.

"*O deus é um!*" A woman in the next row turned excitedly toward me. When I gave her a blank stare, she addressed me in broken German: "Don't you know what you are saying? *O deus é um*—it means 'God is one.'"

Now, I was even more confused. "It's Portuguese," she explained. "I'm from Portugal. I needed to hear that right now— thank you . . . you don't speak Portuguese?"

"Not one word."

A chill went up my spine. *God is one. The Lord is one.* That was the *Shema Yisrael.* Perhaps, *I* was the one who needed to hear it.

When I told Nicole what had happened, she gave me a copy of the New Testament to read. I was particularly fascinated about the reference to speaking in tongues and wondered if this was what—on a small scale, of course—had happened to me. I became even more confused.

There was one section, however, that caused no confusion. It was a section I needed to reread to make sure that the image, which had originally struck me when I had tried reading the New Testament as a young girl, was really there: the woman with the issue of blood. Frantically, I scanned the pages in search of her. Sure enough, she was there, just as I remembered. When she touched the garment of Jesus, he did not recoil from her. This was astonishing behavior for a Jewish man at that time, considering the taboos surrounding menstruation.

According to rabbinical law, when a woman is bleeding vaginally, she is considered "unclean." No one can even take a piece of bread from her hand—not even her husband—or sit in a chair where she has just sat. And this is not only during the time she is actually bleeding but continues for seven days thereafter! Until, on the seventh day, she is cleansed in the *mikva,* or ritualistic bath, she is unclean. An entire section of the *Mishnah*—the oldest part of the Talmud, which serves as documentation of the "Oral Law," or practical interpretation of the Biblical law—takes great pains to delineate the "dos and don'ts" surrounding the menstrual cycle. Even today there are ultra-orthodox Jews who still observe these laws.

For a man to not only refuse to cringe from this woman, but to actually address her, to tell her that by her faith, alone, she had been healed, was moving beyond belief. I was fascinated by this. The simple interchange opened my mind to Christianity, for by this single act, this man named Jesus had done more for women's liberation than any modern feminist ever could. He had treated this pariah as an equal.

This led to my thinking about the prospect of Jesus, the man, as God. What a concept to think that God could love and value woman enough to want to come through her, to be born of her? What greater homage could God pay to his female creation than that? How unclean could this blood be if God himself had been willing to pass through it to experience human life? As a Jewish woman, this was a concept I could not fully grasp, but I liked it.

Of course, it had never really been a question of "cleanliness" at all. In a society without modern plumbing or refrigeration, where people often slept with their animals, what was a little blood? The truth was that the blood was intimidating. At least, what it symbolized was intimidating. Because they could not comprehend it, these men feared its power, so they decided to rob women of this power by teaching them to fear it, too. Why women were stupid enough to listen, I wasn't sure, yet I knew it was surprisingly easy to be swayed.

I, too, recalled being ashamed of my body as a young girl. When I had my first period, when I looked down and saw the blood for the first time, my legs turned to jelly, and my body shook in fear and awe. I was confused, mystified. I was afraid to tell anyone—even my sisters—about my period. In fact, I concealed it, washing my bloody clothes in private; until, one time, when I was visiting my aunt, I was very tired and draped my blood-stained underwear on the back of a bedroom chair, forgetting to wash them right away. My aunt found them and asked me about the blood, and then, everyone in the family knew. I felt disgraced, but I did not know why.

In any event, I became connected on some level to Christianity, thanks to the hemorrhaging woman. She had reached out to me even before I knew that I would one day, thanks to endometriosis, become her. . . .

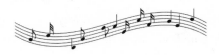

As I studied the Apostle Paul's writings, my confusion returned:

A man should not cover his head, since he is the image of God and reflects God's glory; but woman is the reflection of man's glory. For man did not come from woman; no, woman came from man; and man was not created for the sake of woman, but woman was created for the sake of man. That is the argument for women's covering their heads with a symbol of the authority over them (1 Corinthians).

This was in direct opposition to most Jewish services, where a man covered his head with a yarmulkah, and a woman did not. The Apostle Paul stated that if a woman refused to wear a veil during services, she should have her hair cut off!

Paul's subordination of women was completely contrary to Jesus' example. Why did Paul not learn from Jesus? This was just another example of how all traditions had their warts, and how one should not throw out the baby with the bath water. So why had I done that with my own teachings?

The mysticism of Jesus healing this woman of her painful hemorrhage compelled me to dig more deeply into the power of the spirit, specifically, into the power of Jewish practices in the spirit. Yet, I was a little too stubborn to start with the obvious. I pulled my book on the *Zohar* from one of our many boxes of books and tried to read it again. At this stage of my life, this version of the major text of Kabbalah triggered more frustration than anything else. It was too abridged, too fragmented. I needed to read the real thing—or as close to it as I could get.

This turned out to be no easy task because the author, Spanish mystic Moses de León, wrote his tome in a convoluted brand of Aramaic, constituted by creative grammar and invented words. There were, therefore, only two translations of the book in its entirety in English, and one of them, which had to be ordered from a research center in New York, was over fourteen volumes and cost a small fortune.

There was another, much older, translation done by Harry Sperling and Maurice Simon in 1934, in five volumes, which was, therefore, much more manageable. But to find a copy of it! I was determined, but after talking to countless bookstore owners, librarians, and sundry New Agers in "the know," I was no closer.

Then, one day, I saw an ad for The Strand bookstore in New York City in a metaphysical magazine. The ad actually listed some of its "rare finds"—used books that were difficult to find—and their sale prices. One of these happened to be the very *Zohar* for which I was searching! I called The Strand to confirm that yes, indeed, they still had the books. They were willing to ship them to me if I first sent them a check for three hundred dollars.

Now, even though I knew this was important, three hundred dollars was a lot of money for us at that time. They would not negotiate with me over the phone and halfway around the world, and I had an uneasy feeling about overpaying for a set of books in an unknown condition.

I prayed about the situation, and two days later, an amazing synchronicity occurred. Xao, as part of the small group of Bern Symphony musicians who sometimes toured as the Chamber Players, was going to play a concert in New York! Naturally, I asked if he would mind stopping at The Strand for me to see if my books were still there. He graciously agreed.

When he returned to Bern, he presented me with a set of five immaculate books, neatly bound together by a piece of black string.

"You won't believe what happened!" he said excitedly. "I walked in and asked the man if he still had the copy of the *Zohar* you wanted. He told me that, no, it had already been sold. Well, I was disappointed for you, and the store was really uncomfortable—too warm and dusty—but then, something compelled me to have a look around. Well, I had barely completed an aisle when this high shelf, off to the side and almost to the ceiling, caught my eye. Upon this shelf was a tattered box, positively freckled with holes. Through one of the largest holes, a splash of bright green beckoned to me—but I had no idea what it was. I asked the clerk about the box, and he told me that it was the reject bin for books waiting to go on the clearance rack. I asked him to pull the box down for me, and he reluctantly agreed. When we unearthed the splash of green, we discovered that it was not one book—but five, tied together with this bit of black string. I took the stack from him to look for the titles, and do you know what I saw?"

"The *Zohar!*" Paul and I responded simultaneously.

"Right. In plain white letters, shaded in black—that's what I saw. The clerk had no idea why the books were in the reject bin or why they had come up in his system as sold, but since they were on their way to clearance, he sold them to me for fifty dollars!"

I nearly fainted.

Paul reached into his wallet and pulled out 120 Swiss francs—about one hundred dollars. "Hey man, take this for your trouble."

"That's okay," Xao responded. "I'll just take half—to cover the cost of the books; I was happy to help."

Needless to say, I was pretty excited. The *Zohar* was purported to have so much power that people could be healed just by touching it or by having it waved—like a magic wand—over them.

Yet, the text, itself, was quite a struggle: talk about not having to make sense. Nevertheless, I persisted, knowing that there was power in the words themselves, knowing that my subconscious could absorb the meaning even if my rational mind could not. I struggled to go beyond that rational mind—it was such an obstacle.

Then it was time to move to Vienna and begin my degree program, so I had a forced break from this world of abstractions. The obsession with practicalities that ensued turned out to be healing. I made my goal of getting out of the wheelchair before moving to Vienna, and I attributed much of this to the power of my heightened spiritual life, including the *Zohar*, even if I no longer had the time to actually read it.

After the adjustment period of returning to school was over, I resumed my mystical studies. One night, while poring over the *Zohar*, a passage struck me:

> *When those fools see someone in a good-looking garment,*
> *they look no further.*
> *But the essence of the garment is the body;*
> *The essence of the body is the soul! ...*
> *So it is with Torah.*
> *She has a body:*
> *The commandments of Torah,*
> *Called 'the embodiment of Torah.'*

And later:
The wise ones look only at the soul of Torah.
In the time to come, they are destined to look at the soul
of the soul of Torah!

And later still:
As wine must sit in a jar,
So Torah must sit in this garment.

But of course! The laws, the parables: the *words* were just the garments, the tools—the means to an end. Only fools dwelled on these, wasted precious life debating them. The next level, the rituals, was the body, which gave the garment dimension and shape. Yet, still, this was not the truth. The underlying meaning behind the rituals—what they truly symbolized—this was the soul. Then, "they are destined to look at the soul of the soul of Torah!" Now, the way in which God spoke to the individual through the rituals—and therefore through the initial words—was the "soul of the soul of Torah."

Then I knew what I must do: I must stop looking to the body behind the garments, thinking this made me enlightened. I needed to stop wasting my time trying to find the perfect symbol and focus my energies on what God was trying to tell me through the symbol. Yet, in order to do this, I had, first, to become at least comfortable with the symbol—with the rituals. I needed to go home . . . to Judaism.

It was surprisingly easy convincing Paul to join me in this renewal of our Jewishness, for he did believe that one of the most beautiful aspects of Judaism was the emphasis on the home and the family, and he did so want a family.

"Although it is rather ironic, reawakening to synagogue life in Vienna—the former seat of Nazism," he said.

"Vienna wasn't *the* seat," I responded.

"Well, it was one of them."

To me, such a thought was not ironic at all. It was life-affirming.

We chose Rosh Hashanah—the New Year—as our first service, since this was all about new beginnings.

Rosh Hashanah begins the ten "Days of Awe," which culminates in the most solemn day of the Jewish year: Yom Kippur, or the "Day of Atonement." During these ten days, God is said to open his big Book of Life, judging the goodness of men's and women's lives. Since the actual decision is not made until Yom Kippur, the Days of Awe are a time of penitence, of attempting to start anew.

The synagogue we chose was in the Old City, but the rabbi, himself, was quite young. He was full of energy and ideas.

"'What does God want from me this year?' you ask. He wants you to rededicate your life to him. Do your daily prayers. Spend time with the Creator of the Universe. Are you too proud to do that? If you don't know how, you will learn by doing. If you think spending time with your Creator is boring, perhaps it is *you* who are boring." His face was red, and his eyes were intense. This man was very different from the rabbis I recalled from childhood. I looked around at the congregation. The older members were shifting nervously in their seats, but the young people—and there was a surprising number of them—were hanging on his every word.

"In fact, the only way out of boredom is by communing with your Creator," he continued. "Many of you have become disillusioned by tradition, thinking: 'What does Moses' exodus out of

Egypt have to do with me?' or maybe: 'Why should I shout *next year in Jerusalem* at the end of the Passover Seder? If I want to spend next year in Israel, all I have to do is get on a plane—there's no mystery there.' Yet, these traditions offer lessons for our own time; Jerusalem is only a metaphor: *And I shall dwell in the house of the Lord,* as David wrote. If we do not understand this, we become like Jews around Maimonides' time—the then radical rationalists who rebelled against Spanish mysticism, breaking tradition only for the sake of it—out of ego, refusing to praise God because they rationalized that the Creator of the Universe already knew he was great and didn't need silly, foolish humans to praise him. Such a stance only achieves the opposite of what we desire: we seek freedom, only to end up in bondage. It is not enough just to *think* we are good. It is not enough even to pray—we need to *do* something good!"

I reached out to squeeze Paul's hand, and our eyes met: I knew that he knew what I was thinking: it was not only important to be good, but also to be "good for something." Edgar Cayce's applied spirituality—the final building block to health. It was almost frightening how the wheel kept stopping at the same place.

I also recalled the passage from the *Zohar* about garments and the need to look beneath them. This rabbi was saying that the history—that the rituals!—were the bottle, not the wine. They were only the vehicle to the truth. They were symbols of the *Sefirot,* or levels of God, as were the prophets, as was Jesus . . . or Buddha.

The Kabbalists believe that God is an incremental series of levels, that there are many aspects to the divine personality. Perhaps different aspects of that personality are appropriate for different people. Perhaps that simply changes from country to country, region to region, or even, within an individual's own lifetime. Perhaps a Jew today will need to be a Buddhist in ten years, or vice versa. Perhaps no one is wrong as long as they are *entheos*. Perhaps that is why judging others is a sin. . . .

That night, I had an intense dream: I dreamt I was being crucified. I was taken up to Calvary with a cross on my back. I was kicked and beaten. I was stripped naked. The nails went into the bones of my feet, and I could feel my bones splitting. The pain was excruciating, so excruciating, it awakened me. Yet when I awoke, the pain was still there. I looked down at my feet, and they were gnarled and bent. There was blood oozing from the front of my ankle. The pain was so bad and so odd that I didn't know what to do, so I prayed. At first, I thought I was having some sort of neurological attack, that perhaps my foot had convulsed violently, banging against the bed post, drawing blood. But then, why hadn't it awakened Paul? Maybe my pain was just a vehicle to . . . something else. Maybe it was just the power of suggestion . . . or maybe not.

I pulled myself out of bed and went into the next room to read my *Zohar*. The page opened automatically to the following:

I do not rely upon a son of divinity, but rather, on the God of Heaven, who is the God of truth, whose Torah is truth, whose prophets are truth, and who abounds in deeds of goodness and truth.

There it was again: there is never only one symbol, one way. The Torah was equal to the son. I read on:

When Adoshem wants to bring healing to the world, He strikes one righteous person with disease and affliction; through him, the Holy One, Blessed Be He, brings healing to all. How do we know this? As it is written: "He was wounded because of our sins, crushed because of our iniquities . . . by his bruises we were healed" (Isaiah 53:5).

Hmm . . . So suffering had value—so there *was* such a thing as disease that wasn't self-imposed? I could see why many people believed this passage from Isaiah referred to Jesus: it certainly fit, but perhaps it referred to countless people of no name who had died to "detoxify" the planet. Perhaps it referred both to Jesus *and* to them. The existence of the night does not belittle the day.

Well, all this seemed to suggest that we Jews did not *need* Jesus as the Messianic sect insisted. Jesus was a symbol of the way. Yet, God was many aspects. The Christians confined these aspects to three, while the *Sefirot* of the Kabbalah consisted of ten. Ten made a lot of sense, for ten seemed to be a number of significance. Why were there ten Commandments? Why did the *minyan* require ten men?

Either way, there was clearly more to God than one aspect. Then why did we say, "The Lord our God, the Lord is One?" I believed that "One" stood for unity. God is all things, so He is the unification of all things. In this way, He is One. It was just another symbol—just as my dream had been a symbol.

We need symbols, I thought, *because God wants us to trust Him— to exhibit faith.* If everything is first created in thought—as I learned that night, onstage in Bern—then, of course, none of this magnificence truly exists until we can conceive of it.

I recalled from one of my biology classes that thought processes create a physical path in the brain, in the same way that water flowing in the same direction eventually forms a riverbed. Well, it was my theory that the practice of rational thought by sequential generations had actually created a hereditary physical brain pathway, rendering many of us physically incapable of perceiving miracles. We had simply evolved past them.

I definitely believed that cellular memory existed, for why else would the children of Holocaust survivors exhibit higher rates of cancer and other autoimmune diseases? I, too, was a product of this. My father and a handful of his relatives had barely escaped extinction by the Nazis. Many—including several of his brothers and sisters—had not. My aunt had been brutally gang raped by a group of Nazi soldiers, suffering fatal internal injuries, while my uncle's testicles had been removed—without an anesthetic—as part of the Nazi's notorious medical experiments. Still others had been gassed or sent to the ovens. In addition, my mother was a survivor of the Nagasaki bombing. So, if there were such a thing as hereditary toxicity, I had more than my share. . . .

Although I had the window seat on this flight, there was nothing to see but darkness. I looked over at Paul, who was sitting next to me fast asleep. The book he had been reading—Kafka's *The Castle*—was hanging halfway off his seat, supported gingerly by his dangling hand. Any moment now, the thick book would crash to the floor, waking many of the other passengers who were struggling to grab whatever sleep they could. Carefully, I grabbed the book by the spine, freeing it from its awkward position. Paul stirred a little but did not awaken. *Yes, that's my Paul! Who else would read Kafka on an airplane?* He looked so handsome sleeping there . . . gosh, I loved him.

We had been delayed at airport security because my canes had set off the metal detector, and I could not walk through the gate without them. The guard had been both confused and rude, demanding that I walk through without my metallic canes. Finally, he had let me use Paul as my cane. . . . *How apropos,* I thought—considering to what extent Paul had become my support, buttressing the wall of strength I had erected against the outside world.

I took the small pillow from behind my back and placed it against the window, so I could lean my head against it. Even though I was already several days into my cycle, I still felt terrible. My periods were long—minimum of seven days; sometimes as many as ten; sometimes they even required intervention, such as cauterization, vaginal packing, or ergotrate in order to stop. My pain was still pretty bad, although I was no longer experiencing the "animal pain" of the first two days. Ah yes, Nadja's description was still apt, for the pain reduced me to my most basic, primitive, raw level of being. Luckily, I was beginning to level out emotionally. It certainly seemed that since I had developed MS, an unpleasant synergy had occurred: PMS made my MS worse, and the opposite also seemed to be true. Sometimes, my PMS symptoms extended into the first day or two of bleeding, which I had been told was rare—until I began talking about these things to other women and discovered that it was not so rare. Nonetheless, this had never happened before MS.

Most people's perception of PMS was three days of crabbiness. Well, my PMS was a lot more than that. It often lasted two weeks and caused deep paranoia—and self-hatred. I blamed myself for everything that went wrong. I hated my anger, oversensitivity, and neediness, and it seemed the more I needed people, the more I pushed them away. The hole inside me felt gaping—the loneliness was so great—I could not fill it. It was like a huge cavern, separating me from the rest of the world.

During that time, I also experienced problems with my heart, including an irregular beat, shortness of breath, and chest pain. Even my gums were affected: I would develop several-inch sores across my gum line that were painful and bloody. I also tended to grit my teeth when I was premenstrual, which further lacerated my over-sensitive gums and sometimes triggered an attack of trigeminal neuralgia, which is the most excruciating pain, along the jaw, past the ear, and over the eye. Everything became dark—my life, my looks, my work. I felt fat and useless, unlovable. My cognitive problems worsened, and I frequently could not understand what people were saying. So, I either asked them to repeat themselves, which made them angry, or I simply got it wrong, which made them angrier still. I felt so sensitive that it was difficult to walk down the street, to go among people, for their eyes upon me felt invasive, jagged as bright, afternoon sunlight after exiting a movie theater. To touch someone, to even brush up against her by accident, felt like slivers of glass cutting into my skin.

When the bleeding finally hit, it was like a train wreck: it flattened me, breaking my body apart. The pain began intensely as a huge fist, twisting my insides, and the intensity only grew until it felt like knives, peeling my uterus like a grape: slowly, arduously. I became a deep melon, scooped out bit by bit—roughly, vehemently. My uterus became a caldron of evil; its brew of poison mixing, simmering, gathering in pungency, until it overpowered all other flavors; it's blackness wiping out all other colors.

Needless to say, I knew this was hard to live with, but Paul did a pretty decent job of it. Nonetheless, sometimes, he really pushed my buttons.

For example, there was this one night that he kept bringing up, even though it had happened—gosh, probably a couple of years before, I think . . . well, maybe a year before. Anyway, he was always telling people that I stormed out of the house for no reason and wandered around the city all night, leaving him to worry himself sick about what would become of me. He always made himself sound so innocent. But I remembered what had really happened: all I was doing was trying to practice, and for no reason, he slammed the book he'd been reading on the coffee table. I mean, he slammed it hard! Then he stormed over to the piano and said, all irritable-like: "Give it a rest, already!"

Well, I could see he was in a grumpy mood, so I just figured he had a bad day or was worried about his schoolwork or whatever.

So, I dismissed his insults. Then he started shouting without provocation, and I told him to stop shouting at me. However, he denied shouting at me. Actually, he did that quite a lot: raise his voice to me and deny he was doing it; then blame me for trying to start an argument by accusing him of raising his voice!

In any event, he practically slammed my fingers under the piano lid when he pulled it across the keys while I was still playing. Finally, I said to him: "Honey, if I try, I'm not going to break," and he said: "You're already broken!" Wow! That really hurt. I tried to point out to him that I simply had to use whatever brain I had left, and if that meant going back to school to change careers, then that's what I would need to do. He refused to hear that, so I left the flat for a few hours just to give us a little distance from the situation. And that was it! Nonetheless, he insisted on making a federal case about how self-centered I was.

Another thing that really hurt was that he often took my memory lapses personally. He took offense if he had to repeat something he had told me yesterday or the day before—like I was doing it on purpose, like I was just not paying attention to him. When we were in the throes of the move, I announced a eureka moment: "I just realized that not only is it helpful for me to write everything down that I need to do, but I also need to make a list delineating the logic of my list!"

Well, he became very angry and said: "We spent two hours yesterday figuring that out—what's wrong with you?"

"You know what's wrong with me," I replied flatly.

Oh, well. In the end, the discovery of one's soul mate is not a final destination. It is only the beginning. It is about looking at your own imperfections through the other person's eyes and growing beyond them, together. Although you cannot find your soul mate until you complete your own soul, the appearance of him or her is not a reward, but simply a more powerful impetus to reach your next level: "soul of the soul." To find your soul mate is to begin to find God. . . .

As the dry, cracked land of the desert gave way to a series of mountain ranges—sandy brown to rocky to snowcapped blue, I knew we were getting close. We soared above the Cascades and Lake Washington, turbulence increasing, anticipation mounting. My ears popped like mad, and my stomach felt queasy.

At last, our wheels touched down, and everybody clapped. Were they showing appreciation to the pilot—or just grateful we were still alive?

The pilot responded by announcing: "Welcome to the Pacific Northwest," and my stomach sank to my knees. This was one place I had never been, and it seemed so far away from everything I had ever known. I knew my life had changed forever, yet again.

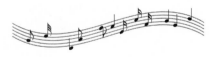

At my in-laws, I sat on the terrace, overlooking Commerce Bay in Tacoma. Stationary ships lit the water like fireflies in the night sky. I could smell the dampness from the rain-drenched rooftops. Smoke rose from behind the stucco middle school, perpendicular to my in-law's humongous condo, making the school look like a Castilian castle in a Greco painting. It was 6:00 a.m., 3:00 p.m. by my body clock. We had arrived late the night before, and I was the only one awake, snug in a silk robe about four sizes too big for me that I had taken from the guest-room closet, which was actually just the overflow of my mother-in-law Karen's many possessions. I felt like Madame Butterfly, sitting in her mother's kimono.

Admittedly, I had enjoyed admiring my thin figure—the only physical attribute I was actually proud of—in the myriad mirrors Karen seemed to require. I played the lady of the manor in my head, marveling at all her feminine accoutrements: the mirrors, make-up, bags of jewelry hung in some kind of system I couldn't figure out but knew existed. I wondered what it would be like to be so gentle with oneself. How would I live with the guilt? I had read *Dark Night of the Soul* by St. John of the Cross on the plane, and I strove for that "separation from the sensual." I longed for the "divine union with God" so much, yet the beauty of this place reminded me that I still longed for a beautiful life.

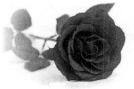

chapter 23: DAWN-PAUL

March 27, 1994

And when the souls are created, male and female are within them together, as one. Later, when they descend to this world, they are separated from each other, the male from the female. The Holy One, blessed be He, reunites the separate male and female soul into one again. It is in their passion for each other that the two souls become one again.

And the Holy One, Blessed be He, created man and woman; two halves of the same whole, he created them, and then split them apart: therein lies the faith.

"You feel so good against me, come closer!"

"Is this close enough?"

"No—it will never be close enough."

"Your lips are so soft. . . . It's so hot in here."

"Well, your body's like a little motor: it generates heat. I could fry an egg on your ass. . . ."

"Yeah, well . . . yours, too."

"The Seder was so wonderful tonight—so powerful."

"I agree. I felt so connected to the symbols—the bitter herbs, the lamb, the salt water, the matzoh . . ."

"The wine . . ."

"Yeah, that, too."

"Well, I felt connected *through* the symbols—to you."

"I understand. You are my temple: through you I have come to God."

"You've always been a person of God."

"I only thought I was—I had no clue."

"This is as close as we can get to God, right here—like this."

"This energy, the center of creation, I've never felt it in this way before. What's happening? I think I'm dying."

"If you're dying, then so am I."

"I think we're—"

"—leaving our bodies!"

"Yes! How did we do that?"

"The energy, what else?"

"But we didn't even try?"

"Of course we did . . . didn't you want it?"

"Yes—I wanted to be closer."

"Well, the last time I hugged you, I projected rays of energy into you, pulling you closer, through my flesh."

"I can see you—you're light! You're layers of crimson, blue, and white."

"Well, you're all orange and yellow . . ."

We are light and sound, brightness and darkness. We are taste and touch: sensing, knowing. Blurring lines of ego, melting into one. Pulse. Severed halves can be re-fused if you accommodate the edges.

Yet, in so doing, we implode into the ache of God. Like the wick on a stick of dynamite, once we're ignited, there is no turning back. Once we are created, we are created forever.

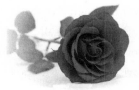

chapter 24: DAWN

April 1994

This is the nucleus . . . after the child is born of woman,
the man is born of woman.
—Walt Whitman

Early spring in Seattle can be rainy and cold. I was sitting at the kitchen table that April afternoon, wrapped in one of my Paul's heavy cardigans, watching the rain turn our small yard into a muddy, sloppy mess. Even in Seattle, rain like this, that lasted all day—sometimes for days on end—seemed to save itself for that raw, restless space between winter and summer.

Three out of the four seasons, the wind blowing off Puget Sound brought rain nearly every morning as chilly temperatures trapped the clouds within the enclave of the city; however, the midday sun could usually be counted upon to give the clouds enough heat to rise over the mountains, providing clear, crisp afternoons that almost never became too hot. In summer, it rarely rained at all.

I think when people talk about how dank and depressing Seattle is, they must have been here in the spring. This spring marked the completion of the first four-season cycle I had spent in Seattle—and the spring was definitely the worst . . . and the wettest. During the past month, the rain really got to me. I had also been so tired that as soon as I came home from my job—teaching at the Seattle Waldorf School—I slumped into a chair, from which it was difficult to extricate myself.

Yet, on this particular afternoon, the dreariness could not dampen my spirits. In fact, the rain was almost soothing. Soft. Vulnerable. Inevitable. Like a baby's cry, it was all in the perception.

I swished a tea bag around a big yellow mug, more interested in feeling the warmth on my hands than in drinking the tea. Feeling sick, I had hoped the tea would settle my stomach. It seemed to have the opposite effect. Nervous butterflies fluttered above the nausea. I waited for Paul to come home from work. Paul, who never complained about the rain.

But after all, Paul had grown up in Seattle—which is why we were here in the first place.

I heard the key in the lock, followed by the sque*eeee*ak of the front door. (No one could *ever* sneak into this house!) Looking up from my dark brew, I met Paul's eyes as he rounded the corner of the foyer. He looked tired. "Hi, Hon," he said through a faint smile. He scanned my face then quickly added: "What's wrong?"

"Nothing's wrong. In fact, everything's right . . . I . . ."

"Wait," he interjected. "Let me grab a cup of coffee."

While he poured a cold cup from the automatic drip and set it in the microwave, I felt like I would burst with impatience. The 'wave signaled a job well done, and Paul removed his coffee—

being none too quick about it, I might add—and sat across from me at the table. I grabbed his hand.

"Paul, I . . . we . . . I . . . am going to have our baby . . ."

At that moment, the tiredness vanished from Paul's face, and his eyes softened. Then his eyes began to dance. Somehow, he looked at me with an expression of both boyish awe and protective pride. No man had ever looked at me that way before—not even Paul, the last time I was pregnant. Something had changed between us: we were now closer, more connected. I could never have anticipated the feeling his expression gave me. I wanted to remember it always.

"When did you . . . but why didn't you tell me it was a possibility?" He stumbled over his words.

"I found out for sure this afternoon. I wanted to wait until I was sure. . . . No use building false hopes—again. Besides, I think you had some idea. . . ." I winked.

"Come here, you minx!" He jumped up and pulled me toward him, then slid to the floor like he was too weak to stand. He kneeled in front of me and gently pulled my legs apart to move as closely to me as possible, nestling his ear against my abdomen.

"Yep, I can hear him in there—or her. Don't want to be accused of giving my daughter a complex!" He laughed as he turned his head to kiss my still very flat belly. "Hey, little one, we've waited for you for sooo long. . . ."

And it was true. Despite everything that had transpired—or perhaps because of it—three years had seemed like a dreadfully long time.

Even now, it seemed like a miracle. Last December, I had found out that I had a luteal phase defect. This meant that in the critical second-half of my menstrual cycle—the luteal phase—

my uterus refused to prepare a home, inviting and comfortable enough to convince a potential child to stick around . . . presuming that my body even produced an egg that month in the first place, which had been determined to be a pretty rare occurrence. My hormones turned out to be even more ineffectual than I had thought.

This had seemed like a good time to try a product that I had been researching for a while: natural progesterone. Since my ability to "manufacture" this secondary female hormone was impaired and my blood levels were singularly low at the wrong times of the cycle, I clearly needed a boost. My research had revealed that synthetic progesterone—or progestins—actually disabled the body's natural hormone production, thereby, in the long run, making the deficiency worse. Research also suggested that progesterone actually assisted in the production of myelin— the very tissue that MS attacks. So it made perfect sense that a woman with MS would have a progesterone deficiency and therefore, PMS, endometriosis, and a miscarriage! It all made perfect sense. Whether the deficiency caused the MS or the other way around, I figured it couldn't hurt to run interference wherever I could. One of my MRIs had shown lesions in the areas of my brain that control involuntary functions, such as hormone production, suggesting that MS had been the initial culprit—and yet, what if I had been born with a hormonal imbalance or had developed one very early in life? It was impossible to be sure how deeply rooted the imbalances were. In any event, it didn't matter. After all, whether you destroy the chicken or the egg, sooner or later, you'll run out of omelets!

The one problem with the progesterone was that my breasts, swollen to twice their normal size, became so sensitive that pulling a sweater over my torso made me grit my teeth.

Why was it so difficult? I had always presumed I'd be a mother—after all, I was raised in an ultra-traditional family—but there had been no desperate, burning desire within me to have children, regardless of the circumstances. Not until Paul, anyway.

Somehow, I had always known that, for me, it would take a very special man. I couldn't have a baby with just anyone—just for the sake of having a baby. It was too cataclysmic, too huge, too magical—too brutal . . . too frightening. I knew that I would have to love someone deeply to transcend the physicality of it. If I had never met that person, I would never have been a mother—simple as that.

But I did meet him. The best part was that, underneath our roles as husband and wife, we were each other's best friend. I had no doubt that I wanted to remain his best friend for the rest of my life—and his lover and . . . the mother of his children. And I knew how very, very much he wanted children.

I stroked Paul's black, slightly thinning head of hair with one hand and wiped my tears away with the other. "I'm going to need you, Hon," I whispered. "I know I talk tough, but I'm really not—I mean, yeah, okay, I guess I'm pretty strong—inside . . . but I'm also terrified. I don't want you to be relegated to passing out cigars. Promise you'll be strong for me . . . promise you'll hold my hand and get me through it. . . ."

"You can bet his—ehh, *her*—life on it."

Needless to say, with my misgivings about conventional doctors even in the face of disease, the prospect of turning the reins of this natural process over to them was not appealing. My idea of the optimal birth experience had always been a home birth assisted by a midwife. For me, the opportunity of learning to transcend pain without artificial intervention, coupled with the freedom to trust my own power—my own womanness—was worth sacrificing technological back-up. I wanted to own my own experience.

Unfortunately, mine was not exactly a low-risk pregnancy: besides MS, my bout of rheumatic fever as a child had left me with a damaged heart valve, which might prove to be a concern. To top it off, there was my proclivity toward bleeding.

With a little persistence, I found a nice compromise: a birth center with all the comforts of home, under the auspices of a hospital.

Other than the aforementioned concerns, my pregnancy was pretty uneventful. I didn't gain much weight, and my doctor chided me about dieting (which I wasn't). I definitely did a lot of swimming and walking, though (these days, I was using only one cane) and yoga in an attempt to build up my stamina. At least, the tingling, numbing pain in my limbs that had intermittently stalked me for years seemed to disappear. The beauty of being pregnant with MS was that actually *being* pregnant triggers a remission of MS symptoms. Carrying a child interferes with an over-defensive immune system. Since, if one's immunity continued to act as paranoid as it does in MS, the woman's body would simply kill the child. Too bad that the downside to this was that childbirth—or the subsequent change in hormones—could often make MS much worse (at least, temporarily). This could make having a new baby even more difficult.

Paul and I had been through this once before, so our eyes were open . . . which certainly didn't make the prospect any less worrisome.

One thing the pregnancy did not improve was the fatigue! My limbs felt filled with sand: who knew it was possible to feel this tired? After enduring, head-on, the brutal fatigue of straight MS, I was now nearly flattened by the introduction of this new mixer: baby. Sometimes, it took me over an hour just to psyche myself into taking a short walk; yet, I was afraid if I stopped exercising, I would never have the strength to make it through the labor. What would it be like? I wondered. Terrifying images from movies I had seen—and even more gruesome self-created scenes—swirled through my mind. What would it feel like to have the baby push through me? Would it feel like ripping? Would the pain really be the worst I had ever felt? My curiosity was answered soon enough.

During the night of December 1, I was awakened by pains in my lower back. They felt like a powerful fist, yanking me to attention. I was concerned because this was happening more than three weeks early. The due date of our baby was actually December 25—Christmas Day. I had been feeling the pains off and on since early afternoon and for the past several hours had been able to sleep through them. I couldn't do that anymore. I picked up Paul's watch from the nightstand to time the contractions. Soon, the episodes were accompanied by a tightening in my stomach.

Paul lay with his back toward me, sound asleep. *I don't need to wake him yet,* I thought. *It's early. So far, I can handle this. Ugh!* Just as the worst pain, up to that point, tore through me. I gasped involuntarily. Grabbing the top patchwork quilt from the bed and a book, I lumbered off to the living room to fight my private war. Needless to say, I couldn't understand much of what I read, but the act of reading kept my mind focused. For the rest of the night, I alternated between struggling to read and walking through miles of living-room rug, until—about a half-hour before the alarm was due to sound—I fell against the couch with a groan, barely able to stand against the pain. My legs shaking, my body bathed in sweat, I stumbled to our bedroom and collapsed against the bed in another contraction.

"Paul!!!"

Paul shot up, confused and dazed. One glance at me, however, and he became unbelievably focused. "Dawn! Oh, God, you look so pale. . . . Are you all right?"

"I . . . think so. I've never done this before. Something tells me it's supposed to feel like this." I laughed as sincerely as I could. "I think it's time to go." At that moment, I felt a gush of water between my legs.

Throughout the long day, Paul was there for me: rubbing my back, telling me how much he loved me . . . holding my hand. The wave of pain rose higher and higher, repeatedly misleading me into thinking I had reached the zenith of my endurance—only to kick up the bar yet another notch. I was awed by my own threshold—frightened even. How could I turn back from this? It became difficult to comprehend an end—that anything had existed before this pain. I sank deeper and deeper into the venerable abyss of it, virtual cycles splicing and re-splicing my awareness: pain . . . until, finally, there was nothing else—not even Paul.

The displacement remained—the disconnection—until voices urging me to "push!" brought me back to a place of tangible control. I found Paul again: he was still holding my hand . . . he had tears in his eyes. He moved to support my back.

"Hold on, my love, you can do it!" The realization hit home that I was crying, too. I mustered all my strength—but our child was in no hurry to be born. Finally, after more than two hours of pushing, I heard myself fully cry out for the first time in over thirty hours of labor. At 7:10 p.m. on December 2, our son, David, was born.

I had made it without drugs or medical intervention—except for some oxygen at one point—and it *did* feel empowering. Our son had pulled out the frightened girl within, along with his life. As I stared at him, lying on my belly—is he *real?*—I heard the midwife say that I had lost an unusual amount of blood and needed to be moved to the hospital. Then I started to hemorrhage in earnest. . . .

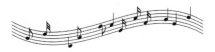

One of my ovaries had ruptured and had to be removed. This, coupled with the extensive endometrial growths throughout my pelvic cavity, several of which had also ruptured during the birth, would—according to the surgeon—make future conception next to impossible. On the other hand, he was amazed that I had been able to have this baby. Nonetheless, due to the risk of hemorrhage, he advised me not to have any more children. "In the unlikely event that you *could* conceive again," he added.

But for now, this news only mildly saddened me because David was so beautiful. When we were making wedding plans, Paul and I had originally dreamed of a family of three or four—but we also knew how fortunate we were to have a child at all. David did require an incubator due to his premature status, and it was extremely difficult not to be able to mother him right away—but the experience only hit home the fact that David was our miracle baby. . . .

Seven weeks later, David seemed to be doing fine. He was not vivacious or boisterous, but I took this as a blessing . . . because I wasn't so fine. In fact, I felt ill most of the time. I had excruciating pains in my left eye and jaw, dizzy spells, and numbness in my left leg. Strange, sharp pains gripped my hands, which felt like they were two-hundred-pounds' worth of thumbs. I struggled to change my son's diapers and to fasten tiny straps.

Paul and I had agreed that I would give up working full time to stay at home with our child for at least the first three years of his/her life, so I had planned to leave the Waldorf School at the end of the first semester, right before the holiday break. I had felt so unwell by Thanksgiving that work had become a real challenge. However, when David made his appearance early, I couldn't complete the term anyway.

Originally, I had planned to balance freelance assignments with the care of our child, but now, my fatigue was so great that I doubted my ability to properly care for our son at the exclusion of everything else. What happened to my empowerment and newfound confidence? A sense of failure settled in and remained my constant companion.

One night after dinner, while sitting on the living room floor, fumbling with my leaden hands to sew David's ripped sleeper, I broke down and cried bitterly. "I don't know what's wrong with me, Paul," I sobbed. "Everything hurts; I am so, so tired; my hands don't work. I feel like an old lady! How am I going to do any work? How am I even going to be a good mother to David?"

Paul sat down next to me on the floor, his hand reaching up to stroke my face. "Don't be so hard on yourself, Hon. David doesn't look like he's wanting for care. . . . You had a hard time . . . you lost a lot of blood. The doctor said that alone could give you a longer-than-average recovery. That's all it is. You've got to learn to pace yourself—take a nap when David does. . . . You didn't really expect to take on freelance projects right away, did you? We agreed to make sacrifices financially to give our child the right start. . . . You're not impatient with that already, are you?"

"No, of course not," I said rapidly, growing defensive. "David is my number-one priority. I just feel so bad!"

"You know, there is something else," Paul began tentatively.

"Yes . . . ?"

"Well, the MS—I know you don't like to dwell on it—but you know we talked about it. MS sometimes gets much worse after giving birth. . . . You may have to accept that. Look what happened after the miscarriage. You are doing so much better than you did then. If you need extra help right now, we should address that. Getting depressed is not going to help."

"I'm not depressed!" I snapped. "This is the happiest I've ever been in my life . . . if only I felt well enough to enjoy it!"

"It's just going to take some time," he said, kissing my forehead. "Look, I know you probably don't want to hear this, but it really might be a good time to see the neurologist. At least, you'll get a clinical assessment of where you are."

The neurologist did not offer much more encouragement. In fact, he suggested that I stop breast-feeding, in order to go on Betaseron, which was now available to the public. This, I refused, and resigned myself to returning home quietly to resume my struggle without further complaint—lest I be manipulated into subjecting my body to more powerful toxins and their often-debilitating side effects—not to mention, depriving our baby of nature's head-start immune-builder: his mother's breast milk. Besides, with or without MS, I didn't like the idea of admitting that childbirth—a natural process—could actually kick me on my ass.

Nonetheless, months went by, and time did not make it all go away. In fact, things only got worse. I began having episodes of falling: my legs would just give way beneath me, like the scene in Disney's *Bambi,* where the fawn attempts to walk on the frozen pond. (My speech had become peppered with such allusions now that David was relating to stories and pictures!)

By now, Paul was quite concerned, and he had nearly convinced me to stop breast-feeding and start the Betaseron. It was a bit too late, however, for two nights after our talk, I suddenly and completely lost the vision in my left eye. A spidery, almost electrical pain seized my skull. It felt like a bucket of ice water, laced with jagged little knives, had been dumped on my head. The shakes began: until I couldn't stand anymore. I flung against the couch grabbing my head. I couldn't breathe. At that moment, I felt like I was going to die. I don't mean I "thought" I was going to die—I mean, my body actually had a physical sense of inevitable danger. "Oh, God! Paul! [gasp] I think [gasp] I need to go to the hospital . . ."

Paul looked up from the dining room table, where he was writing out bills. He waited a moment, then walked—calmly—to the sofa. "What—what is it?"

"My left eye . . . blackness . . . nothing . . . I have [gasp] the strangest pain . . ."

David began to cry. I suddenly noticed that the left side of my body had disappeared. "I can't [gasp] move my left side."

"Dawn . . . *Honey,* can you hear me?" His voice trailed off in my consciousness. I could see him picking up the phone. Everything went black.

I was hospitalized for a week of IV steroids to stabilize my condition. I felt like a big dope. But then, it was over in a few days; I *did* feel quite a bit stronger, and I could go home. I soon found plenty of new worries to keep my mind off MS. . . .

It was not difficult to see that David was not a normal little boy. He was weak and slow, and he tired very easily. He seemed to be short of breath and had difficulty eating. He certainly did not compare with the rambunctious handfuls that were my friends' six-month-olds. Even with my MS, he seemed to tire as easily as I.

"He's just mild-mannered and cerebral," Paul said. "You'll see, he's a runt, but he's strong! He takes after you." Nonetheless, I could hear the masked worry in his voice.

One night, David awoke with a bizarre fit of crying. It was an eerie, awful sound—not so much crying, as struggling for air. Struggling in pain. His cries stopped and started like a flap was opening and closing in his throat. As he lay in his crib, his skin shone blue against the white sheets. His body felt limp like a rag doll. I picked up the phone to dial 911, but before I could get through, Paul had already scooped up David and was headed for the door. "The hospital's five minutes away this time of night— we can do better ourselves. Let's go."

Time stood still within the walls of the hospital. Too exhausted for rational thought, too terrified to speak, we hung by, limp as useless appendages, while the wizards in white coats ran high-tech tests on our tiny baby. Our bleary eyes were glued to these figures of hope—the only power in this strange world— darting back and forth.

Finally, after what seemed like lifetimes of stale anguish, held down by sips of bad coffee, the head wizard spoke. Our worst fears were realized. David had aortic stenosis, which meant the valve leading to his aorta was too narrow to allow blood to flow freely from the left ventricle of his heart to his aorta—thereby hindering blood flow to the rest of his body. His heart muscle already showed signs of thickening, and his ventricle was enlarged. He required a catheterization as soon as possible to stretch his aortic valve to permit blood to flow through.

I was too numb to speak.

Paul assumed his take-charge stance. "But how did this happen."

Dr. Wizard: "Aortic stenosis is one of the most common forms of congenital heart defect, which means your son was born with it. In most cases, there is no known cause as to why the heart fails to develop properly inside the womb. Sometimes, it's genetic, sometimes it comes from exposure to certain medications during the first trimester of pregnancy . . . sometimes, it happens when the mother drinks alcohol while carrying the child."

I did not take offense at this, but Paul did: "My wife did everything she could while carrying him." For a minute, I was afraid that he was trying to convince himself, and that hurt. "She didn't even drink a single glass of wine after she found out she was pregnant!"

The doctor appeared almost amused, which seemed strangely incongruous to the situation. "As I said, *most* cases are not associated with any particular cause. The last thing we want to do is assign blame."

Paul looked away.

"It is important for you to understand that time is not on our side," the doctor continued. "Your son's aortic valve is nearly fused shut. His heart stopped briefly in our examination room—he had to be given adrenaline to start it up again. If we wait even a few days, I am concerned that acid will build up in his blood, and his internal organs will not be able to receive sufficient blood supply. There is already slight hemorrhaging into his lungs. Valve replacement is too risky right now—due to his condition and his size. This will be a viable option down the road—perhaps a mandatory step . . . if he survives. The catheterization is our best bet. Again, considering his current condition and his size, I cannot promise you that we will be successful—but it is our only hope . . ."

I suddenly found my voice. "Are you saying that our son could . . . *die* from the procedure?" I met the doctor's eyes without mercy.

He met my gaze for a moment, then looked away all too quickly before he spoke: "Yes. At least, he could die, *despite* the procedure. Without the procedure, he most definitely *will* die."

My legs began to buckle beneath me, and my cane clicked against the linoleum floor. Paul grabbed my arm.

Paul: "Just tell us what we need to do to save our son."

Dr. Wizard: "I'd like to move him to Children's Hospital— as soon as possible. There is a surgeon there with extensive experience in catheterizations on infants and small children. We will take care of it. I just have some papers for you to sign."

Two days later, we held hands in Children's Hospital, praying, while surgeons threaded tiny wires, encased in plastic tubing, through our son's veins and arteries, into his heart. The wires guided a deflated balloon into his aortic valve, which was then inflated, ripping open the fusion to give renewed life's blood to his struggling little body.

The surgeon emerged. "It looks really good," he said simply. "Looks like he's going to make it."

A handful of words that gave us back our lives. At least, for a time . . .

A few short weeks after the procedure, David seemed like a different baby. He brimmed with energy. His curiosity and his movement wore us both out. We relished our hope. We dared to plan.

Nine months later—when David was fifteen months old—an attack, much worse than the first, sent us back to Children's Hospital for another catheterization. Again we hoped.

"It is, unfortunately, quite common to need to repeat this procedure," the surgeon told us. "The valve just fuses up again. You need to be aware that there comes a point when catheterization ceases to work. That's when the valve, itself, must be replaced."

We knew this was probably inevitable, but at this point, we just wanted to buy time until David was older and, hopefully, stronger. We just had to make sure he grew older.

Then, one month after his second birthday, David was frolicking around, tormenting his father like any normal two-year-old, when he suddenly collapsed. His breathing was a hollow, haunting sound.

Oh, God, please save our son!

We knew what was coming. When the doctor spoke, it was an empty formality. "We must replace the heart valve. As time is not on our side, we need to go with a mechanical device. I know you both are quite familiar with the risks involved, but there is no other option. We will do what we can."

Before he went back to work, the surgeon paused to touch my hand—a flash of his humanity. For a moment, I saw not a wizard in a white coat, but a man. A man who allowed himself to grasp, for a moment, what a woman was feeling while her child lay dying.

"Paul, look how little he still is," I whispered to my husband as we stood next to our son's bedside to pray before the surgery. The ventilator groaned. The sheets drowned him, so all you could see were a small limb here and there, pieces of boyish face—and mounds of plastic. I couldn't control the tears, as much as I wanted to stay strong for David in case he *could* see me. "How can his tiny body endure this?"

Without looking at me, Paul began to sob. . . .

The biggest problem with mechanical valves is that they have a tendency to form clots that can break off into small chunks, spraying like flak into the circulatory system. These *emboli* can lodge in the brain, causing a stroke.

This is precisely what happened to our little boy, following his valve replacement. Forgive my bluntness, but this lack of drama has been my only means of surviving this. He remained in a coma for eight days before renal failure set in, and he died.

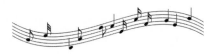

Although Paul and I needed each other more than ever, we had never been more distant. It was jarring to discover, after so much we had shared, how differently we each dealt with something as basic as grief. I felt it should be a private pain: no one outside our marriage could feel this in the same way, and I didn't want to include them beyond the formalities. I felt the best thing Paul and I could do was to give each other space within this space—and just be gentle with each other.

Paul, on the other hand, needed discussion. Although we had always lived rather privately, self-contained, he suddenly needed more people around. He began bringing our friends and relatives into the experience. Hashing it. Analyzing it.

I had believed in preserving my heart and passion for one man—my husband. Paul had, therefore, received all my passion, all my heart without reservation. It was painful to hear him say: "How can you believe in God after what happened? No God would do that to our son. There is no God. . . . After everything we went through, how could David be taken from us?"

My grief, strangely, was more spiritual and physical at the same time: I felt a physical ache around my uterus. I had even bled for over a week after David's death. Yet, I also believed the Khalil Gibran sentiment: *Children come through you, not from you . . . your children are not your children.* Despite my grief, I was grateful to have "borrowed" this beautiful being for as long as he was given to us. I knew this was too big to control. Paul needed to be able to control it.

Speaking of control, during this time, I was receiving yet another lesson on how to relinquish it. I began having a type of seizure that disassociated me from reality. The episodes were like being suspended in altered awareness—like a wall had come down between me and the outside world. I was still alive, but I could not connect to my life. My neurologist suggested I have an ambulatory EEG to chart and evaluate the seizures. . . .

As I walked into the examining room, the technician asked me many questions—probably due more to curiosity than to necessity—about my cane, the weakness on my left side, etc. Even to professionals, MS remained a curiosity. Finally, as we reached the room she said: "You don't have MS, do you?"

"Yes," I said.

Her eyes projected a level of compassion not usually seen in a clinical surrounding. Was it for real? I couldn't tell.

I was instructed to lie on a rigid, white-lined cot with my neck supported by a rolled-up towel. She proceeded to mark my scalp in various places with a red pencil, while—again, more for curiosity—asking me questions like: "How long have you had MS? What were your early symptoms? How did you find out you had it?"

I was a little annoyed, for I was here for the evaluation of seizures, not MS, per se.

Tiny electrodes were then glued to my head and sealed with an air tube. It smelled like someone was building a model airplane in my hair. The wet, Crazy-Glue-like substance sputtered into my ears and eyes. The bundle of eight sturdy black wires was grouped at the back of my head, then thickly taped next to my shoulder blade and swung around my right shoulder, between my breasts, across my stomach, and down the left side of my body. Taped with what looked like a bandage in several places, the wires would extend almost to my knee, except that they were intercepted by a hefty recording device that was encased in black and strapped to my waist by a brown belt big enough for a large middle-aged man with a weakness for beer. It reminded me of the belt my father used to "whup" me with when I was a child. The wires met at the left side of this box, at the top of which was a blue button (which I was instructed to push at moments of particular suffering, so as to highlight my brain activity at those times).

To the left of the blue button was a digital clock displaying in military time. I was given a "diary" in which to record—every hour on the hour for the next 48 hours—what I was doing and what I was feeling. If I felt anything particularly unusual between the hours—or did something noteworthy like take a pill or a pee—I was to make a separate entry for that as well. You see, the ambulatory EEG "allows your physician to monitor your brain-wave patterns during your everyday activities such as work, play, sleep, eating, etc." The idea is to see how your brain responds during specific events. In my case, they were looking for evidence of seizure activity.

The main hole in this theory was that—between the device and the wires—it would be very difficult to pursue my "normal activities." For one thing, the recording device measured 5½" x 4½" x 1½" and felt like it weighed about five pounds, which I suppose if you were a 170-pound man, would not be a big deal; however, to a ninety-six-pound woman, it was an impediment. I was already dizzy and weak, so carrying around this hefty recorder did not exactly give me much motivation to "continue my activities." In our technological age—in these days of micro-cassette recorders—you would think they could get the job done with less bulk.

Secondly, I had electrodes, covered in white gauze, attached all over my head—including two very obvious points at my temples—with black wires mangled through my hair like calamari in capellini. They had made me unpin my very long hair from its well-groomed bun at the nape of my neck. Between the glue, their efforts to push my hair aside to get to my scalp, and the fact that I couldn't brush my hair lest I disengage the wires, my head was a mangled mess of stringy tangles. Add to this the fact that I had a large hunk of electrical tape slapped against the left side of my forehead to hold a particularly stubborn electrode in place. Yep, I looked like the Bride of Frankenstein. Also, there was no way to hide this massive recorder strapped to my waist—unless I zipped up a man's jacket and wore it all the time! Needless to say, I wasn't exactly going to the grocery store looking like this.

Therein lay the irony of this experiment: how could they get a handle on my brain waves during normal activities when I couldn't continue normal activities wearing this device!

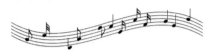

In Your Diary . . . include all your activities, and the time of day, including walking, eating, sleeping, urinating, and sexual activities.

. . . Yeah—like someone would make love to me in this get-up? What planet are they on??

Besides, I have cognitive impairment after all. How am I supposed to figure out this diary? . . .

Before I was sent home to "go about my normal activities," I was given a conventional EEG. I was told to close my eyes, open my eyes about a million times, and then move my eyes without moving my head. I was asked to open my mouth and hold it open, pretend I was chewing gum, and grit my teeth. I was asked to breathe deeply and quickly for three minutes. Then, when I thought I would pass out, the technician started flashing bright lights in my eyes. This was by far the worst part of the test—I felt like a prisoner of war being tormented for information. "I feel like you are trying to extract military secrets from me," I said. "What is the purpose of these lights?"

"To irritate the brain," the technician said. And then, as if realizing how bad that sounded, she quickly added: "Ehhr, to highlight any abnormal responses."

Her first response appealed much more to my twisted wit, and I refused to let her off the hook: "Irritate the brain, huh?" I chided.

I heard her repress her laughter. "Now, now, be serious. . . . I didn't mean that exactly."

"But that's what it is . . . exactly."

The lights burned hot and red, dancing in rapid jumpy patterns. There was more redness than light, and the experience was more than bright lights: it usurped awareness, stretching the visual fields like a taut blanket, end to end—pushing out any other sensation. Even with my eyes closed, there was no escape— it was all there was—no beginning and no end. (From those lights, I was dizzy and nauseated for three days.)

After this, the tech asked me questions to evaluate my cognitive awareness, like: "Who is the president of the U.S.? What is the month? What is the year? Can you spell 'world' backwards?" Then, she asked me to subtract seven from one hundred, then seven from ninety-three, and so on, until she told me to stop. I think I got to fifty-eight.

These were the same questions I had been asked by countless medical professionals for years. Even if I could not do the calculations, I might have been able to memorize the answers by now. Besides, if only my daily life were that simple! How did these infantile questions ascertain whether my cognitive impairment interfered with my daily life?

The hospital was an hour away from my home, and I could not see well enough to drive. Since Paul was working, I took the bus. The minute I arrived home, I noticed that one of my electrodes had become disconnected. I called the EEG lab.

"Can you come back at once?" the voice asked.

"No," I said. "The hospital is an hour away, and I need a ride."

"Well, then, you will have to adhere it to your head the best way you can."

I opened our so-called utility drawer and pulled out a roll of electrical tape. Too tired to cut it into neat segments, I tore off a long strip with my teeth and slapped it across the electrode. I just didn't have the time to compete with Miss America. . . .

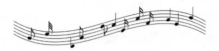

One night we actually decided to do something normal like go out to dinner. It was nice to escape the sorrow of familiar things, to feel life again—or pretend to. I was glad to have Paul, grateful for his love. After a little wine and food, I leaned in, grabbed his hand, and whispered: "I'm going to do terrible things to you tonight, Mr. Bailiff."

He was not amused. "You're rather amorous. How can you be thinking so much about sex now? Is it some twisted effort to have another child?"

"Why would that be twisted?"

"Well . . . considering we can't."

I sighed and looked at him: "I just need you so—I need your touch, I need to feel, I don't know . . . flesh—life inside of me. I need to feel *you* inside of me. Tell me I'm beautiful . . . tell me how much you love me . . . tell me how much you want to make love to me . . ."

"I do love you and yes, you are beautiful . . . but I can't make love to you right now. I'm too tired. I have too much on my mind. I'm sorry."

When I awoke the next morning—Sunday, his day off— Paul was gone. He didn't call. He didn't come home until after midnight . . . and he was very drunk.

"Where have you been?'

"Nowhere."

"Why didn't you call?"

"Get off my back."

"I was just—concerned."

"Oh, so it's fine for you to go hit the bars—but not for me!"

"What bars? I had two glasses of wine at a family tavern."

"Oh, whatever—I'm going to bed."

The next morning he was too hung over to go to work. Even though I was still angry, I felt sorry for him; so I brewed him a cup of herbal tea, took it into the bedroom, and handed it to him without a word.

"Thank you," he took the cup from my hand, smiling sheepishly, apologetically—gratefully.

"It's okay."

"Look, I'm sorry about last night. I just needed to—be alone with my thoughts."

"I said it's okay." And that was that. I was hurting, too. I didn't have the strength.

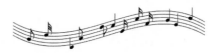

Paul withdrew more and more from me, deflecting my love for him.

"I miss you," I said nestling close to him, putting my hands on his face. Grabbing my hands in mid-caress, he said simply: "I can't."

We spoke no more that evening. Then, in the middle of the night, I was awakened by Paul kissing my back. He pulled me close, and I could feel him hard against me. He turned me on my back and began sucking my breast. Despite my tiredness, my body responded to him. I had ached for him for so long—I began to encourage him along. Without giving me enough time, he thrust himself into me. He was rough and forceful. He had never been that way before. He had made love to me with gentleness, respect. Deep force had always been painful for me, due to the endometriosis, and it had become even more painful after David's birth and the subsequent surgery. Paul knew this. It was something he took care not to do. It did not matter this time. I gasped in pain. My body became rigid against him.

"Paul, please! Why? It hurts so much."

He pretended not to hear me. After becoming satisfied with taking his rage out on me, he pulled away abruptly and sat on the edge of the bed, his back to me.

I felt violated, expendable, meaningless. I bit my lip to keep from sobbing. It worked. "What was that?" I asked with only ice, no emotion.

Paul opened the nightstand drawer, took out a cigarette, and lit it. He had just recently started smoking. "Isn't that what you've been nagging me for—a good fuck?"

Pain and rage exploded in me like a flare. I grabbed his arm and turned it hard, forcing my nails into his flesh, forcing him to look at me. "I have been *offering* my *love* to you, hoping you could express your love to me. At least, it used to be love."

I could no longer hold back the tears, and I left the room without looking at him. There was a futon in David's room. I would sleep there—when I could sleep. Right now, I could not stop crying.

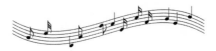

A kiss on my forehead and the smell of coffee pulled me out of sleep. Paul was sitting next to me. He handed me a hot cup. He looked worried, recalcitrant. Through my fog, I could not tell if he was sincere.

"I . . . don't know what to say about last night. . . . I am so sorry, of course. . . . I'm sure that doesn't mean much, right now. I can only hope and pray that you can forgive me. You didn't deserve that . . ."

I wasn't ready to speak.

"Well, come on and have some breakfast," he said.

"I'm . . . not . . . very hungry." I sat the coffee down.

"C'mon," he urged, pulling me to my feet. "I made pancakes. . . . You'll feel better after you eat."

We ate without speaking. Every once in a while, he paused to touch my hand. I stiffened instinctively to the gesture. I struggled to swallow past the knots in my throat.

Finally I spoke: "Paul, why do you hate me?"

"Hate? That's a strong word."

"Well, why do you resent me then? What is it that you think I should have done that I didn't? Why do you blame me?"

"Blame you? That's ridiculous."

"It's not ridiculous that you want to hurt me."

He dropped his fork and sighed.

"And it is not just last night—though that was the most obvious. You have been cold and withdrawn to me since right after David's death. This morning is as attentive as you have been to me in weeks—and that's only because you're guilty." I thought he would become angry then, but he didn't. He just looked very, very sad.

"What can I say? You're right," he said quietly.

That stung, but at least we were making progress. "Can you tell me why?"

"You've been so insensitive to my feelings, lately; I guess I've grown insensitive to yours."

"What is *that* supposed to mean?"

"You figure it out."

"I think you blame me because I can't have any more babies—and the one I did have was too 'inferior' to live! That's what I think! But how can you blame me for that? It's not my fault! I did everything I could to have a baby—and a healthy baby. But the cards were stacked against me. Damn it! Could it have been any more difficult and painful? Now, suddenly, I feel that you've 'dismissed' me—like I'm no further use to you!"

"Honey, no—God, how can you think I could . . . I am so proud of you. You are so strong . . . sometimes, just too strong."

"Meaning what?"

"Meaning it's okay to ask other people to do things for you that you no longer can."

"I don't understand. We've been through this. Adoption for a disabled woman is next to impossible."

"I want another child."

My eyes began to burn. "But what can I do about that? . . . I can't."

"But I still can."

"What?"

"Well, what about surrogate mothers?"

Frankly, the idea of another woman having my husband's child was too painful to bear. "How can you bring that up to me now? When you know how much it hurts me?"

"Maybe I just wanted to see if you can still feel pain. I wouldn't know that from your reaction to David's death. . . ."

I was dumbfounded. I knew we were crossing into the land of "you can't take it back," but I couldn't let it go. "God, Paul! How can you think this doesn't tear me up? I was his *mother!* I carried him inside my body, for God's sake!!"

Wrong thing to say.

Paul's eyes flared: "What? Don't you think I would have carried him if I could? Why do women have to resort to statements like that? Don't you know how privileged you are?"

Ouch. Yes, I did, but somehow, I had always guessed the forced pain of the privilege excused a little knife twisting. I suddenly realized, for the first time, that it did not.

"Look, Paul, I didn't mean it like *that.* . . . Okay, maybe I did. But it was a low blow. I'm sorry. But how can you even think that I'm not grieving David's death, just because I handle it in a different way than you do? How could you hurt me like that?"

His eyes softened. "You're right. That was an atrocious thing to say. I'm sorry, too. . . . I guess I just need some time to adjust to the fact that it is going to be you and me from now on—and that is it."

I walked over to him and gently put my hand on his shoulder: "We need to learn to live with each other again without the distraction of a child."

Again, wrong thing to say.

He flared again: "*Distraction?!* Is *that* what he was?"

Now, I was too hurt to speak. Paul had stopped taking his medication, and he was not thinking clearly, but still . . . Paul knew I had been a good mother—that being a good mother meant everything to me. When did I become the enemy? Suddenly, I didn't know this man who stood before me. Somehow, a lifetime between us was gone. I don't know how, but it was.

Paul spoke, more quietly this time. Eerily. "He was—the only son I'll ever have. It's the death of a dream. I can't just walk away and say 'life goes on.'"

But by now, I was too hurt for compassion. "Well, look on the bright side," I snapped. "When I'm dead, maybe you can get remarried—to a *healthy* woman—and have more children!"

He shot me a look of pain. "Considering what we've been through together, that's a hell of a thing to say."

"This conversation is full of those! Why stop here? How do you think what you said made *me* feel? Like you just married an incubator. I know it's my 'fault' you won't have any more sons. What can I do about that? I love you! You are the only man I could ever imagine sharing that with. I would have ten babies with you if I could, despite all the pain! Giving birth to our son was the most amazing thing I have ever experienced—painful, yes, terrifying even, but empowering, expansive—complete love, which the word 'love' doesn't even begin to describe! That feeling that brought us together is still here! It didn't die with David! God, Paul, are you saying that everything you felt for me was based on a dream, on the future and what *could* be?"

"I don't know what I'm saying. . . . I don't know anything anymore. . . . I know I don't want to hurt you . . . but I need to figure this out without worrying about repercussions."

Fear, emptiness rose in my stomach and choked my breath. "Paul, what *are* you saying?"

"I've always admired your strength—but with strength comes coldness. And I can't live in the cold—not anymore. If coldness is what it takes to survive, then I don't want to survive. Coldness is just the other side of stopping in a way—it's just an illusion . . . it's . . . ."

He continued on, in this mad way. I no longer saw a man in front of me—only the inner little boy. And I still loved that little boy. I put my arms around him, and, for a moment, he just hugged me and sobbed.

"Oh, God, how can I say this when I know how much it will hurt you? How can I say this without ripping myself into pieces, since we're one and the same . . . I . . . *have* to have more children. I can't help it; I need another child. . . ."

I pulled back, frozen. My soul felt diced into tiny pieces that sliced my insides each time I dared move or take a breath. I felt dizzy, faint. I grabbed my jacket from the back of the chair.

"Paul . . . I . . . don't know what to do with that. . . . I need some . . . air. . . . I'm going out. . . . Please don't follow me."

I stumbled into the night air as from a painful, violent dream. I wandered the streets in a daze. When I grew tired, I sat on a bench, a step—whatever. Then, I kept on walking. I have no idea how long this continued.

When I finally returned home, the house felt different somehow. Strangely still. I guessed Paul had gone out to think things over as well. I needed to sleep. I headed for the bedroom. The stillness seemed to grow somehow, suffocating me as I walked. I felt I was going to vomit. I slumped weakly against the bed—my body gave way against the hard edge of the mattress, very much like it had over two years ago when I had come to tell Paul our baby was on his way. Now, however, I was weighted by anguish—without destination . . . without end. This time, Paul did not wake up to catch me. This time, Paul lay on the bedroom floor with a gun in his hand. And a bullet in his head.

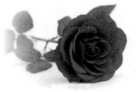

chapter 25: DAWN

July 1997

Paul did not die right away. When the paramedics arrived, he was still breathing, so he was taken to the hospital. I rode in the ambulance. They said it was critical, and if I wanted to say goodbye, I should do it now. He was receiving blood and morphine. One of his eyes was completely destroyed, and the other one was closed. He did not respond to my voice. I touched his hand—it was warm but unresponsive.

When we arrived at the hospital, I just sat there and held his hand. The rabbi stepped in and told me that hearing is the last sense to go, so "be gentle with him."

I was annoyed by this, but merely responded peacefully: "Yes, I know."

I had nothing to say accept "I love you"; nothing else mattered now. I held his hand for the six hours he had left. I didn't even leave to use the bathroom. When I tried to pull away, his fingers would close around mine as though he didn't want to let me go. I hoped he knew I was there—but I didn't really think he did. His fingers reacted to touch—but it was more automatic than kinesthetic, more reflex than response. I knew this because when I tried coming at his hand from different

315

angles with my finger, his hand tightened in exactly the same way each time. . . .

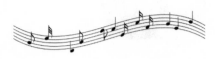

My face hurts; I am cold; my brain is surreal. I am not sure what that means, but I don't have to know: it is *my* brain. I am fighting my body. My back and neck hurt, and my face pain is intense, radiating from my jaw to under my eye and into my temple. I feel grumpy and resistant. I feel like I can barely exist let alone create. How can I justify my existence? I have become so less of myself, so incomplete. The misery ties me to my body, and I wander inside like a widow inside an empty house: lonely, confused, knowing I should do something with what is left but not being able to muster the strength. Oh, wait . . . I *am* a lonely widow. I don't need metaphors; my life is colorful enough. I want only to sleep—if the pain would only let me. . . .

I don't know how to live an experience without owning it; how do I change quickly? Either way, I am alone. Now I have no choice but to lean completely on God, and therefore, myself . . .

MS put me in touch with my physical self—a facet I have long denied in favor of my mind. When I became sick, my body cried out louder than the unwillingness to surrender ever did. To release control—that's always the hardest part . . . and the most important: of music, of illness, of love . . . of God.

As a classical musician, I learned to muffle my body's outcries—against exhaustion, stage fright, hunger, jet lag, pain, and loneliness. Now I have to listen to heal—I have to relax into it. I have to reverse years of instilled discipline. The greatest bravery is trust.

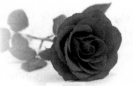

chapter 26: DAWN

January 2007

Where does he wander,
I wonder,
My little one,
Hunting dragonflies?
—Chiyo (18th century Haiku poet,
written after death of her young son)

After the loss of my husband and son, I was forced to look only to myself for healing and survival. In so doing, I needed to face what many solo women come to realize: despite the women's movement, we are often still marginalized in society to the point of suppressing our own true identities. To be a woman should not mean that we need to be less of a human; however, this is often the case. Sometimes, this is our own fault because, in our attempt to find equality, we wear hats that hide our faces.

Although it seems liberating to discard the veil, we must be careful not to be distracted by the milliner's pretty colors. We must be careful not to exchange one mask for another.

Five years ago, I was diagnosed with ovarian cancer. I was told that *with* treatment—which consisted of a complete hysterectomy, followed by chemotherapy and radiation—I had an "80 percent probability of expiring in three months or less." The doctor did not offer any alternative to this rigid protocol and strongly urged me not to consider surgery without the follow-up chemotherapy, even though he admitted: "the benefit of postsurgical therapies in advanced cases such as yours is not well-established."

So, the medical profession could offer nothing besides the "unholy trinity" of surgery, radiation, and chemotherapy, which had no real precedent in cases like mine and, at best, only promised to buy me a few months.

The vivid memory of my aunt, weakened and disfigured by chemotherapy agents, dying of ovarian cancer anyway, made me reluctant to follow his advice.

Despite having two of the risk factors—familial tendency (both my aunt and grandmother had succumbed to the disease) and Jewish ancestry (Jewish women are stricken in disproportionate numbers)—I was not diagnosed until it was "too late." The so-called screening tests for ovarian cancer are deemed "unreliable" and are, therefore, not covered by insurance.

Besides, the symptoms of ovarian cancer—abdominal and lower back pain, bloating, bowel problems, nausea, and irregular vaginal bleeding—are similar to those of endometriosis, which I have been battling for over twenty years.

As my attacks of painful bleeding became increasingly life-threatening, I was, at last, referred for a battery of gruesome tests, including culdocentesis—a procedure in which fluid, removed from the area around the ovaries via a needle inserted through the vaginal wall, is analyzed for the presence of cancer cells—and transvaginal color flow doppler—a type of ultrasound in which a plastic probe is inserted into the vagina to measure both the resistance and the speed of blood flow to the ovaries. (Since malignant tumors require an increase in blood vessels, which afford little resistance, a less inhibited blood flow suggests their presence. Even benign growths, like ovarian cysts, do not interfere with the normal functioning of blood vessels.) The surgery that followed—both diagnostic and debulking (the "hollowing out" of as much tumor mass as possible)—was as far as I was willing to go.

Not only did the degradation of hysterectomy/chemotherapy/radiation not seem like a worthwhile trade-off for short-term survival, but the removal of the center of my womanhood was not a concept I could accept. It was not only a question of slamming the door on motherhood once and for all, but of altering the very core of what made me who I was. Of course, I would still be female sans a few organs, but would I still feel like a woman—at least, what my body had taught me being a woman was supposed to feel like? I had never denied that my hormones shaped the way I thought, felt, and interacted with the world around me. Without them, who would I be?

How strange that the medical profession is so quick to rob women of their womanhood, that even feminists—who are supposed to champion all that is woman—often view such identification with one's ovaries and uterus as a sign of oppression. After all, what man would deny that the loss of his testicles would jeopardize his manhood? Even the very thought makes most men cross their legs. Why should we, as women, be any less possessive of the very things that make us who we are?

Sometimes, one must "die by the sword" not because of karma, but because she has lived with the sword for so long that ceasing to be a warrior would be more painful than ceasing to be.

A key problem with such bravery is that it is difficult to find role models: truly strong women who are unafraid to embrace their femininity. We claim we no longer believe that rational thought and intuitive emotion are mutually exclusive; why do we live like we do? Who says that power has to be aggressive and explosive? It takes just as much power to be patient and enduring.

My healing process has encompassed the physical and the spiritual, the alternative and the conventional, bringing me to the conclusion that there is no "good" or "bad," but merely what works and what does not. The soul can only understand absolute value; it passes no judgments. Only the mind does that. Only the mind looks for comparisons.

When I was a girl, I thought Ayn Rand was a role model. After all, she was certainly a successful woman—*Atlas Shrugged* had sold more than any book other than the Bible—and she was rational. It was only much later that I realized the illusion of this: Ayn Rand and her idolization of Aristotle—Aristotle who taught that a woman ranked slightly above a slave but nowhere near the status of a man. Aristotle who, along with Plato, recommended female infanticide as state policy.

Ayn Rand and her living of the rational life—what does a woman like her have to teach the ordinary woman? She was completely disassociated from her womanness. As Nathanial Branden wrote in his book, *Honoring the Self:* "Ayn Rand was the father I never had."

Personally, I would rather listen to a woman with five children talk about her day. There is more wisdom in that.

When are we going to value the true wisdom, the power, of motherhood? I have accommodated another being inside of me, taken my husband into me and felt his energy, his cells, grow into a separate, glorious creation. I have become one with that being's hiccups, movements, restlessness, and fear. And it has become one with mine. I have faced death to send this being into life, staring down the dark corridor of pain the way a man stares down the barrel of a gun in battle. But there was no glory in my battle, no medals or decorations. Because I am just a woman, after all, and this is what I was created to do. Babies are born every day. My bravery remains unsung because it is built from quiet things like love and pain.

People talk about being brave enough—or having a high pain threshold or loving someone "enough." But if you talk to the "bravest" people, they say that they just did what they had to do at the time without thinking. They did not get up one morning and say, "I think I'll be brave today." When discussing the experience, they will usually tell you they were terrified. If you do what you must do, despite the fear, that is bravery.

Love comes out of the day-to-day struggle with a person—not from some huge emotion that hits you out of nowhere. It is in the quiet moments, in the so-called little things: in making tea, in listening to a dream for the two-hundredth time, in cleaning the toilet, in wiping up vomit.

The best way to deal with great pain is to dive right into the middle of it—like an ice-cold pool of water—and let it envelop you, carry you. If you resist, you tense, you tighten, and create even more pain. The pain is there—no matter how you resist, you cannot change that. Yet, it is an involuntary, human reaction to withdraw. One must focus on the smallness of being, on the essence. This is why the Lamaze method works so well. The smallness of breath. When the mind tries to encompass the entirety, it freezes. Repetition of one small truth is far more effective than the study of hundreds of complex koans. This is also why the rosary works. In the smallness of a simple prayer, one finds acceptance and the courage to also remain small. Like the willowy reed in the Aesop fable, smallness gives one the malleability to embrace pain. In the embrace of pain lies empowerment.

And yet, the world would rather look to men who kill and conquer, who *inflict* pain as examples, or to women like Ayn Rand who trivialize their female power, who seem ashamed of it, who strive to develop the masculine within themselves. This is a more comfortable image for society: the glorification of the masculine, the suppression of the feminine. The blood still engenders shame. The menstrual shelter has become invisible, but it still exists. Until we stop concealing our blood and pain within the confines of the Red Tent, we, too, will remain invisible . . . and we will remain sick.

Seventy-five percent of all autoimmune diseases are suffered by women, and this figure is growing. According to a new study by the U.S. Department of Health and Human Services, between the 1980s and the 1990s, the proportion of women living with multiple sclerosis rose 50 percent, while the proportion of men living with MS remained constant. Autoimmune diseases like MS are the result of the body attacking its own tissue. They are maladies of repression, of anger and frustration turned inward— maybe even of self-hatred. If we are so "in tune" with ourselves as women, if we are so "liberated," why do we have such a need to self-destruct? . . .

These are my thoughts today as I light the Yortzeit, the memorial candle, on the tenth anniversary of my son David's death. These are the things I have learned—and also my distractions. In all this time, I could not bring myself to visit David's grave. I could not face the reality of my little boy being no more. How could I accept that the body I had carried in my body and had known so well—every hair, every dimple, every imperfection that somehow seemed perfect—was now in the ground, where it would remain? How could that be him? How could it no longer be him?

Although I have always believed that the body is little more than a shell to house the spirit, my mind cannot grasp the idea of the body simply ceasing to have significance. This body that, throughout our time on earth, continuously cries out for attention—to be fed, washed, groomed, loved.

At the same time, I cannot accept that the spirit, once departed, would hover around the body. Why would the person we loved be anywhere near his grave? Wouldn't he have better things to do? I cannot understand why so much emphasis is placed on the grave. Perhaps it's because it's the only *symbol* we have. And, yes, we humans need our symbols, don't we?

I am going to visit David's grave today. The idea came to me in increments—but I pushed them back. It has taken me several hours to leave the house.

As I drive to the cemetery, I get a flat tire. Luckily, I know of an excellent tire shop nearby, so I drive—slowly—to the repair shop. While I wait, I see an ad for Perelli tires. Perelli makes a type of tire that just sucks up nails and keeps going. *What an idea!* I think. *I would love to be able to do that: suck up all the nails in my path and keep going, unscathed.* Or would I? "The unexamined life is not worth living," said Socrates, and he was right.

While some traditions believe that we choose adversity to grow faster, others believe we grow from adversity. It doesn't matter. The point is: sometimes, we must just run flat . . . sometimes, we must live with the questions. No, I don't want to suck up the nails and move on. What I want most is to learn to run flat. I want to avoid "petrification," as Jung put it. I want to accept that oftentimes pain is the most effective path to wisdom or enlightenment. It is not the only way, but it is probably the most thorough.

Perhaps I no longer believe in the perfect soul mate—but wasn't I so much happier when I did?

Perhaps we simply create everything because we need a challenge. Like a small child playing chess with his father, we say to God: "Please, Daddy, don't let me win! I want to be big and smart like you! I want to *really* win! I want to earn it!"

I once heard Dr. Arthur Caliandro speak about grief at the Marble Collegiate Church in New York City. "You must not be distracted from grieving," he said. "You must grieve. You must live into the pain."

That's why I am at the cemetery—to live into the pain.

The sight of *David Bailiff* carved on the tombstone makes me fall to my knees at the foot of the grave. I cannot feel my soul. I vow never to say a mean thing to anyone again. I vow to never lose my patience. . . .

Perhaps even David is my symbol. Through the experience of motherhood I learned that I couldn't do anything more important to connect myself to God than be a mother. Through my experiences as a mother, I also learned to write. In writing, I had to learn to trust my psyche, just as I had to trust my body in childbirth.

After the death of my family, I threw myself into teaching, both at the studio and university level. I needed the children. In addition, the rigors of running my own studio—my own business—kept me occupied. It also kept me from writing. I was afraid to step off the cliff, afraid, in the final analysis, to face the pain of both loving something so deeply again—as I had loved music, Paul, and David—and of confronting my losses. Yet, I reminded myself: the experience of fear does not preclude bravery. So my greatest fear became my greatest healing. In many ways, my greatest suffering has been this book—but it has also been my greatest healing. And in the midst of my greatest suffering, I have realized how wonderful it is to be a woman and how grateful I am to have experienced a woman's pain. Yet, I strive not to become attached to this, for I know that pain, too, is a symbol—of the "soul of the soul." It is the white-hot fire used to forge fine steel from our lives.

I try to feel the pain of my little boy's death—and my husband's death—at this tombstone—but once again, I feel myself holding back. I become annoyed with myself. I know that I will not split in two, that I will not disintegrate and yet, I have too much fear—even to be brave.

I have everything I need in the present moment to come out the other side, intact, I tell myself. Indeed, I have everything I need right in my own tradition, in my own life—and in the lives of all those around me. *The Lord our God, the Lord is One* . . . we are in His image, so we are all one: Buddhist, Christian, Jew, man, woman. There is no division. And because there is no division, the smallest activity is prayer. . . .

I drive to a dollar store and buy two balloons: one with a yellow smiley face and one with a red heart. On the smiley face, I write: David Bailiff, my little smiley, died January 7, 1997. He now flies with God on the wings of my—his mother's—love. On the red heart, I write: Paul Bailiff, my husband, died July 23, 1997—*Dein ist mein ganzes hertz.*

I go to the most beautiful place I know—a big rock perched above a river. I look out over the city skyline. The waters crash over the rocks below. I feel a tremendous power in me that I cannot define—like something is about to break apart. (Maybe I *can* disintegrate, after all.) I say a prayer—or rather, I *feel* a prayer (there are no definite words)—and I release the balloons into the air.

As I watch the wind carry these symbolic souls of the men I loved higher and higher above the trees, the greatest sorrow I have ever felt—a sorrow I previously forbade myself to feel— wells within me, making my knees buckle. The pain is so great I feel it could kill me. Breathing becomes difficult as my vision clouds with tears. There is nowhere to go but up—and out. I release my pain to the universe, feeling myself split open—not unlike giving birth to David—but this time, it is my own soul coming forth. This time, that which I bear cannot die.

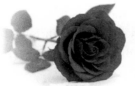

about the author

Fluent in five languages and competent in several others, Dawn Bailiff has worked as both a translator and Internet marketing consultant for *Fortune 500* companies, as well as an academic translator of Rudolph Steiner, G.W. F. Hegel, and Martin Heidegger. She has also been a successful journalist, technical writer, banking officer, college professor, and small business owner. Dawn Bailiff holds an undergraduate degree in music from the esteemed Peabody Conservatory of Johns Hopkins University in Baltimore, Maryland, as well as graduate degrees from the University of Vienna, Austria, in technical translation and philosophy. She is also the author of *Using Music to Teach Math, Foreign Language, and Technical Skills—Incorporating the Anthroposophic Principles of Rudoph Steiner* (written in German).

Ms. Bailiff's most recent translation credit is *Cosmic Ordering: The Next Adventure* by Barbel Mohr (published in May 2007 by Hampton Roads Publishing

Company), and she is currently translating Barbel Mohr's next book, *Complaints to the Universe*, also for HRPC.

For more than a decade, Dawn Bailiff was a world-class concert pianist on five continents, soloing with most of the major symphonies and philharmonics, including Berlin, Vienna, Munich, Prague, London, Tokyo, Chicago, and Los Angeles, with such notable maestros as Leonard Bernstein, Carlo Maria Giulini, Eugene Ormandy, and Sir Georg Solti. At the age of eighteen she toured thirty-two cities in six months, playing in such exotic locations as Bayreuth, Wurzburg, Wroclaw, Istanbul, Hong Kong, and Seoul.

Also a composer, her works have received numerous performances. Her opera, *Anblicke des Himmels und der Hölle* (for which she wrote the libretto in German), was performed in Berlin, Dresden, and Stuttgart.

Both she and her music have been featured on North German Radio (NDR) in Hamburg, Czech-Slovak Radio (CSR) in Bratislava, BBC World Service Radio, CBC Radio Canada, CTV (Canada), YTV (Canada), *Good Morning Canada, A.M. Philadelphia, Good Morning America,* and National Public Radio (WHYY).

As a writer, both her poetry and short fiction have received international acclaim.

A spokesperson for MS and the disabled as well as a performance artist, she shares her experiences with groups as wide-ranging as veteran organizations, women's groups, churches/temples, art centers, bookstores, schools, libraries, and political forums on human rights. She has spoken frequently to "standing-room only" audiences. She also conducts "writing to heal" workshops and is available for bookings as both a speaker and facilitator. Visit Dawn Bailiff online at www.members.aol.com/dawnbailiff.

Hampton Roads Publishing Company

. . . for the evolving human spirit

Hampton Roads Publishing Company
publishes books on a variety of subjects,
including spirituality, health, and other related topics.

For a copy of our latest trade catalog,
call toll-free, 800-766-8009,
or send your name and address to:

Hampton Roads Publishing Company, Inc.
1125 Stoney Ridge Road
Charlottesville, VA 22902
E-mail: hrpc@hrpub.com
Internet: www.hrpub.com